Wellness ConneXion

Simple Secrets of Ageless Vitality

BY

Dan Watts, M.D.

Adrian Lewis, M.D.

Steve Kalishman, J.D.

Foreword by Steve Dailey

The information contained in this book is based on the research and personal and professional experiences of the authors. It is not intended as a substitute for consulting with your physician or other healthcare provider. Any attempt to diagnose and treat an illness should be done under the direction of a healthcare professional. The publisher does not advocate the use of any particular healthcare protocol but believes the information in this book should be available to the public. The publisher and authors are not responsible for any adverse effects or consequences resulting from the use of the suggestions, preparations or procedures discussed in this book. Should the reader have any questions concerning the appropriateness of any procedures or preparation mentioned, the authors and the publisher strongly suggest consulting a professional healthcare advisor.

Published by Wellness Authors, LLC
Wellness ConneXion: Simple Secrets of Ageless Vitality

Catalog-in-Publication Data is on file with the Library of Congress
ISBN 0-9774668-0-9

For information, write

Wellness Authors, LLC
9127 SW 52nd Avenue, Suite 102
Gainesville, Florida 32608
(866) 374-7161

Printed in the United States of America.

Inside text design/layout by Lena Shore

Cover Design by Shaw Creative

Illustrations by Hyun Hee Park

Adrian

*With gratitude and humility to the Lord who has
forgiven and blessed me beyond what I deserve.*

*To my wife Sue, whom I adore, and to our exceptional
sons, Andrew and Mathew. I will spend the rest of my life
striving to be the husband and father you deserve.*

Dan

*In gratitude to my wife Sherry and my two children, Ashlee
and Danny, for supporting me and always believing in me.*

To my mom and dad for supporting me through medical school.

*And to my patients for leading me to practicing
prevention-based medicine.*

Steve

*With gratitude to God for the gift of life and the
ability to learn how to live it abundantly.*

*To my wife of 29 years, Natalia, and my daughter, Sasha, who are
my main reasons for wanting to live 100+ years in good health.*

*To my law office team, Charlene, Dave, Joy, Pete and Roxana,
for covering for me while I pursue my dream of helping
people realize their full potential for ageless vitality.*

And to my mom and dad, who are both in great health in their 70s.

For more information visit our Web site at
www.wellnessconnexion.com

Contents

_____

ACKNOWLEDGMENTS

Like the pursuit of wellness, creating this book was a journey that involved input from many people. Chris Angermann's role in orchestrating this project was invaluable. Susan Angermann, Debbie Baker, Tom Campbell, Steve Dailey, Dr. Jenny Druxman, Robert Ferguson, Elizabeth Hanselman, Matt Kalishman, Dave Lewis, Judith Nagan, Sally Vickers, Sherry Watts and Diana Worth reviewed the manuscript and provided support, suggestions and insights. Connie Crutherds contributed detailed suggestions, as well as her own story, to one of the chapters. Susan Hicks proofread the final manuscript with wonderful attention to detail. Lynn McDonald provided important advice on how to guide the manuscript to publication.

The doctor of the future will give no medication, but will interest his patients in the care of the human frame, in diet, and in the cause and prevention of disease.

THOMAS EDISON, AMERICAN INVENTOR

FOREWORD

Listen to your heart.

If you are an "average" American your heart will beat somewhere between two-and-a-half and three billion times during your lifetime.

Seem like a lot? Think about when your heart will thump its last 500 beats. Or 100. Or 10.

At some point in your life, life itself will be your most dominant, significant focus. Every breath, every heartbeat, every movement of every muscle will be precious.

And the question this book asks is "When?"

When will the next beat of your heart, the clarity of each breath you take, the level of vibrancy and flexibility you enjoy when you move, the confident endurance you feel as you pursue your goals in life…when will these things that are the most precious indications of life itself be your most dominant, significant focus?

Well, if you want the last 10 beats of your heart to be as far into the future as possible…NOW is that time.

Our culture has trained us to address health only when we are "sick." Ironic as it is, mountains of evidence reveal that we don't reflexively focus on health…when we are healthy. Dr. Adrian Lewis, Dr. Dan Watts and Steve Kalishman believe it is time we change that.

The book you are holding is a simple, concise and easy-to-apply collection of insight and direction on how to make the rest of your life the best of your life. You will discover that the definition of health and wellness is not about running around the block in spandex shorts or diving into yet another celebrity-endorsed diet. Health — defined by your authors as Ageless Vitality — is about embracing a balanced lifestyle and monitoring simple, everyday activities that make a dynamic and noticeable difference — for good. You'll discover that good choices based on simple principles and sound, scientific fact can yield remarkable results; and that Ageless Vitality is not just reserved for obscure cultures that feast on mysterious forms of seaweed and water spiked with rare minerals.

No. The picture of lasting energy, graceful mobility and true longevity can be staring back at you in the mirror every morning... as long as you make a decision today to begin to make better choices based on the insights and advice in this book.

A final note before you begin this revealing trek: As you read through the authors' fundamental wisdom presented in the following pages, you'll face your first, defining choice. You'll have a choice to be simply entertained or truly inspired — only casually informed or motivated and moved.

Make the right choice. As you read, take notes. Make some new commitments. Design a plan for how you'll apply what you'll learn. How you elect to digest this book will be the first decision you make among many that will launch you to a fulfilling journey resulting in a healthier, rewarding and more vibrant experience of what life offers all of us if we only decide to embrace it.

Listen to your heart. Every...single...beat...is precious.

Steve Dailey

Steve Dailey is a professional business coach and fitness advocate. He has authored "The 14 Keys to Balanced Health" audio series, contributed to three best selling books on sales success with sales expert Tony Parinello, and published numerous audio programs and eBooks on principles in growing small business. At age 51, Steve continues a lifelong passion for fitness through swimming and bicycling, most recently posting six rankings in the top 10 in the country in Master's Swimming.

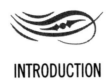

INTRODUCTION

YOUR CONNEXION TO AGELESS VITALITY

---

*If I'd known I was gonna live this long, I'd
have taken better care of myself.*

EUBIE BLAKE, JAZZ COMPOSER, AT AGE 100

The United States is the richest country the world has ever known.
We enjoy unprecedented wealth, opportunities and lifestyle.
Living in a land of plenty, we naturally expect to have the best of
everything. But when it comes to health and healthcare, we are not
even near the top.

We spend nearly twice as much per capita on healthcare as
Australia, Japan, France, Germany and Great Britain, yet we have a
shorter life expectancy and higher infant mortality rate.[1]

More than 60 percent of the population — across all age groups
— is overweight, and nearly one-third of all adults in the U.S. can
be classified as obese. A large number suffer from cardiovascular
disease, breast and colon cancer, and type II diabetes, all related to
obesity. An estimated 300,000 Americans die each year from direct
or indirect causes related to obesity.[2]

Diabetes, a chronic illness with no cure, has become the fifth-deadliest disease in the United States. Its complications include heart disease, stroke, vision loss and blindness, kidney disease, and amputation.[3]

Many people of normal weight are unhealthy, too, suffering from chronic headaches, stomach disorders, body aches, arthritis, depression and many other common ailments. Modern American medicine tells them that these aches and pains are an inevitable part of aging.

More than 46 percent of all adult Americans take prescription drugs daily, many of them for headaches, upset stomachs or other stress-related illnesses.[4] As a nation, we consume almost half of all medications in the world.[5]

How ironic. We spend more money on healthcare than any other country; yet, as a nation, we are overweight, unhealthy, tired and unhappy. For obese people, the emotional suffering may be as painful as the physical aches of their condition. In a society that equates attractiveness and success with being slim — especially for women — overweight people are constantly told in one way or another that they are second-class citizens.

The real tragedy, however, is that many Americans do not realize that a majority of their ailments are simply the result of how they choose to live. They lack basic information to make the connection between lifestyle choices and wellness. Unaware of the link between poor diet and health, for example, they do not understand that there are simple measures that will vastly improve the quality of their lives.

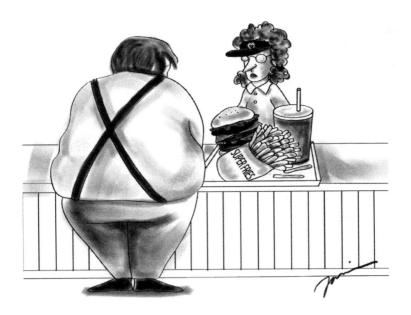

"Would you like life insurance with that?"

There are two groups of Americans that have made the connection and historically pursued a healthier lifestyle — the media elite and the wealthy. In the case of Hollywood actors and other media figures, their livelihood depends on looking fit. Unlike most of the general population, they exercise, undergo detoxification programs, eat healthier food, take nutritional supplements, and make use of all the newest and best developments in anti-aging and wellness research.[6] From Suzanne Summers, looking fit and trim in her 50s, to Paul Newman at 80, many aging celebrities radiate health and energy.

Over the past 10 to 15 years, many young professionals and baby boomers have started to follow their example. But the knowledge of how to improve one's health and wellness, although available to all, has not yet fully penetrated to the general population.

Why Do We Ignore the Obvious?

If the possibility of radically improving the quality of our lives is well within our reach, why do so many of us continue to follow a path that leads to sickness and chronic ill health? There are a number of reasons.

For years, a trillion-dollar food industry has bombarded Americans with messages designed to addict us to a diet of processed and fast food.[7] Each day, the average American consumes the equivalent of one stick of butter! We have become a junk-food culture, eating more fat and sugar than is good for us by any standards. No wonder obesity is out of control!

A steady diet of junk food depletes the body of the essential vitamins and minerals it needs to function well. In the short term, the resulting deficiencies lead to mood swings, lack of energy and joint pain. In the long run, they may cause major illnesses like cancer, diabetes and heart disease.[8]

These illnesses play into the hands of a profit-driven pharmaceutical industry, which often appears more interested in treating symptoms than in actually improving the health of Americans. Drug companies spend more money on advertising than on research.[9] Because it is more profitable to develop drugs that consumers use for life instead of just once or twice, most research dollars go to products that treat the symptoms rather than the causes of disease.

The American model of medicine is very effective in managing trauma and acute illnesses, but it does not work well for chronic conditions that result from diet and lifestyle abuse. Many doctors continue to undervalue the role nutrition and exercise play in health, despite scientific studies that directly link disease and aging to poor food choices and lack of physical activity.[10]

In addition to lack of exercise, medical attitudes, and a profit-hungry pharmaceutical industry, there are other important issues that affect our health and well-being.

The food we eat has become less nutritious over time. Due to soil depletion, processing and growing practices — such as picking vegetables too early, ripening them in vats of gas, and transporting them over long distances before they reach the consumer — it is difficult to get all the necessary vitamins and minerals from our diet. You may think you are eating well, but if you get your food only from traditional supermarkets, you may be undernourished.[11]

Another major issue is the increase of pollutants and contaminants in the water we drink and the air we breathe.[12] Pesticides, gasoline emissions and dioxins are on the rise in our environment. Although the U.S. government has banned some of the worst toxins, such as DDT and polychlorinated biphenyls (PCBs), studies regularly show that our environment is far from safe. DDT has a half-life of 57 years. Environmental pollutants continue to find their way into our bodies.

We absorb these toxins directly from the air, through the food we eat, and from the water we drink and bathe in, storing them in the fatty tissues of our bodies. According to estimates based on breast milk concentrations nationwide, at least five percent of the babies born in the U.S. are exposed to PCBs sufficient to cause defects.[13]

There are numerous studies suggesting a link between these contaminants and the rise in breast cancer, the increase in male reproductive disorders, and the drop in fertility rates throughout the Western world.[14]

What Is to Be Done?

There is good news. In recent years, because of anti-aging research and a better understanding of how our bodies work on a cellular level, doctors and scientists have come to the following conclusions[15]:

- Aging is a natural process.

- Maintaining our quality of life as we get older is often a matter of choice.

- Health science can slow down, stop and even reverse

many of the symptoms that steal our health and rob us of our looks.

- We have the power to significantly influence the length and quality of our lives.

We invite you to take part in these exciting developments. We have coined the phrase "Wellness ConneXion" to emphasize the link between these discoveries and specific applications that will enhance your health and well-being. The "X" symbolizes the intersection of new or definitive knowledge and people wishing to improve the quality of their lives.

The Wellness ConneXion

It would be a shame to squander the best years of our lives having to endure chronic pain, ill health, low energy and depression, especially when we now know that they are not inevitable. Nor is there any reason for most of us to be miserable from age 60 to 110, and to spend the last of our golden years in a nursing home.

The building blocks of wellness are known and can be used by anyone. To that end, we have identified seven interlinking principles that provide the essential "conneXions" for you to improve your health. Some of them may seem simple and obvious, yet they remain a secret for many Americans. We continue to be surprised by the number of people we meet — even highly-educated ones — who are unaware of the essential link between food and well-being, for example.

The seven principles that provide the conneXion between you and the most up-to-date knowledge for a better quality of life are:

1. Pure Water

2. Eating Right

3. Eliminating Toxins

4. Supplementation

5. Exercise

6. Stress Management

7. A Balanced Life

It is our belief that if you make the conneXion, using each of these principles, your health and quality of life will improve significantly.

We know that to maintain our economic lifestyle after retirement, we need to develop a plan and follow it for many years. Many Americans have a portfolio of investments for just that purpose. Why not develop a portfolio to benefit our current and future health?

Some people reject the path to wellness because they believe it is too expensive. They say things like, "I would do it if I had a cook, maid, personal trainer and life coach like Oprah." While we understand that not everyone can afford cosmetic surgeries, unlimited supplements and services that will improve health and looks, we believe that better health and well-being is attainable by everyone. Therefore, we recommend starting small and sensibly, spending a reasonable amount of money and time — say $50 to $100 a month and a few hours a week.

How to Read This Book

What prevents many people from getting started on improving their lives is confusion about where to begin. Every few months, the latest solution is advertised on late-night television. Since the 1950s, the U.S. Department of Agriculture has changed its dietary guidelines numerous times.[16] Considering the glut of diet books on the market, who can tell which ones makes any sense at all?

In each of the following conneXion chapters, we summarize the problems of one major area in which people's lifestyles affect their health and well-being. We outline generally agreed-upon medical and scientific knowledge, as well as the most recent research discoveries, and recommend common sense approaches for your wellness journey. We conclude each chapter with three simple, inexpensive suggestions on how to get started.

The order of the chapters is deliberate. We begin with water, the wellspring of life, and work our way toward the ultimate goal of a balanced life. But each chapter can stand alone. You may wish to read the book quickly and go back to the sections that appeal the most to you, or read the sections that you wish to work on first.

An appendix includes references for those who wish to delve into these principles more deeply, for readers who have already embarked on their journey toward greater wellness, and for healthcare professionals who wish to scientifically verify the recommendations made.

What to Expect

Most chronic illnesses develop over a period of 20 to 30 years. Fortunately, it will not take nearly so long to heal. We believe that even if you practice only some of these wellness principles on a regular basis, you will see significant improvements in your health, energy and joy in just a few months.

John Molloy, a 56-year-old school administrator from Connecticut, became obese when he took on a stressful job and went through a divorce. He started to walk after work and watch his consumption of carbohydrates. Over the next six months, he lost 52 pounds and his blood pressure returned to normal. By making these simple choices he had the pleasure of feeling in control of his life again.

Wellness is not a result but a process, a way of functioning in the world that requires daily practice. Just as good athletes train on a daily basis, and child rearing or a good marriage require ongoing attention, so a healthy lifestyle is a matter of actions repeated on a daily and weekly basis. The way to improve the quality of one's life is to integrate positive habits into daily routines, to find pleasure in eating right, fun in exercising, and joy in balancing one's life.

Americans have a "can-do" attitude. We believe in the possibility of change for the better. We live in an exciting time. Never before in our history has there been such an opportunity for being in the driver's seat on the journey to improve the quality of our lives. For anyone wishing to make personal health and wellness your destination, these conneXions are the road map.

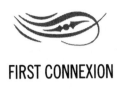

FIRST CONNEXION

Pure Water

There is no small pleasure in sweet water.

Ovid, Roman Poet

Pure, clean water is not only the wellspring of health and well-being; it is a matter of life and death.

Except for the oxygen in the air we breathe, water is by far the most important substance we need to survive. The human body can do without food for long periods of time. Mahatma Gandhi, the father of modern India, protested British rule by fasting for as long as 40 days without suffering lasting ill effects. Had he been deprived of water, he would not have lasted much more than a week.

Nearly three-quarters of the body consists of water, leading novelist Tom Robbins to quip, "Human beings were invented by water as a device for transporting itself from one place to another." Water provides hydration and helps the body eliminate toxins that build up in the cells. Without it, the liver and kidney, two indispensable filters, are not able to perform their essential cleansing functions, and death soon follows. In the words of Nobel Prize-winning biochemist Albert Szent-Györgyi, "There is no life without water."

We in the U.S. are blessed with an abundant supply of water. We can turn on the faucet just about anywhere in the country and have access to drinking water, either from a public water system or a well. By comparison, two in five inhabitants of the globe face a shortage of water.

In addition, much of the water in the world is unsafe for human consumption. The World Health Organization (WHO) estimates that 72 percent of all communicable diseases, including cholera, typhoid and dysentery, are transmitted through contaminated water. The results are often unpleasant symptoms like diarrhea, as tourists in foreign countries often discover, or sometimes even death.

We like to think that we are exempt from such problems in the U.S. We are confident that "Don't drink the water" is necessary advice only for travelers going abroad. Unfortunately, that is not the case. It turns out that the water we rely on, the water that gushes forth when we turn on the faucet, is not the safe, clean substance most of us think it is. In fact, many doctors and scientists have warned for years that drinking tap water is dangerous to our health.

Chemical Pollution

With the development of the chemical industry in the 20th century, pesticides, chemicals and fertilizing agents have become a permanent part of the water supply. They enter groundwater and aquifers through disposal sites, animal wastes, runoff and sewage. According to the Environmental Working Group (EWG), based in Washington, D.C., manufacturers released more than one billion pounds of toxic chemicals into rivers, lakes and other bodies of water between 1990 and 1994 alone.[1]

No wonder a 1999 government report concluded that much of the nation's groundwater and many streams were contaminated with pesticides and dangerous levels of fertilizer chemicals.[2]

Doctors and scientists caught on early to the fact that these chemicals are harmful to human beings, causing cancer, respiratory problems, birth defects and other illnesses. Responding to a mounting crisis, in 1974 the U.S. Congress passed the Federal Safe Drinking Water Act (FSDWA). As the most comprehensive legislation ever enacted to protect water sources and drinking water, the FSDWA set up government oversight through the

Environmental Protection Agency (EPA) to regulate a number of hazardous chemicals and contaminants.

Since then, however, the EPA has set national safety standards for less than 100 pollutants. We use more than 75,000 chemicals regularly and develop over 1,000 new ones each year! As a result, according to the Ralph Nader Research Group, "U.S. drinking water contains more than 2,100 toxic chemicals that can cause cancer."[3]

And that covers only the 250 million Americans who rely on public water supplies. The rest use private wells, which are subject only to state and local laws. Some of them contain considerably higher concentrations of chemicals, because their water comes directly from contaminated aquifers.

Even when hazardous chemicals are banned, they remain in our water supply. DDT, a cancer producing pesticide whose use became illegal in 1972, continues to show up in streams and fish across the U.S., in both rural and urban areas.

The reason chemicals persist in the environment is that the global water cycle is a closed system — no new water is created. It simply keeps recycling from the oceans to the air to rain to groundwater and aquifers as it has done for millions of years. We are using the same water that the dinosaurs did 200 million years ago.

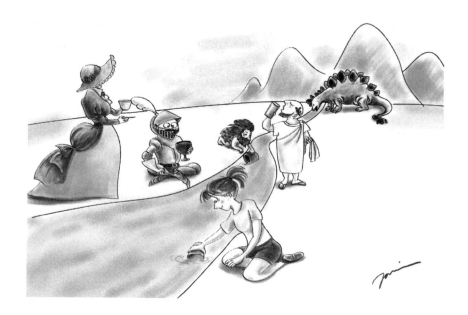

We drink the same water the dinosaurs did.

As a result, whatever chemicals we manufacture — gasoline, pharmaceutical drugs, dioxins, nitrates — find their way into our water supply and stay there, most of them harmful or deadly to human beings.

Lead and Asbestos

Lead is a toxic element that accumulates in the body's tissues, especially in the brain. Over 30 million Americans drink water contaminated with high levels of lead, most of it from old water pipes and solder used in plumbing. According to the Washington Post, more than 250 major cities currently exceed the EPA's lead standards.[4] One of the authors of this book was recently found to have four times the normal levels of lead in his body.

Janice, a 60-year-old post-operative nurse, came to see Dr. Watts, one of the authors of this book, when she started to experience memory loss and tremors. She was worried about getting Alzheimer's, and embarrassed when she could not control her trembling hands at work. Tests revealed that she had high levels of lead in her body, in all likelihood caused by the plumbing in her house. She had inherited her childhood home, along with its old lead pipes, and continued to live there. On Dr. Watts' recommendation, Jeanie installed a water filtration system and underwent detoxification. Soon the tremors disappeared, her mind regained its sharpness, and she had more energy than she had ever experienced before.

Lead is particularly dangerous for infants and children, who absorb more than adults, because they drink more water in proportion to their body weight. Many studies have documented a relationship between lead and hyperactivity, attention deficit disorder and drops in IQ levels.[5] An EPA Report summary states, "Each year in the U.S., lead in drinking water contributes to 480,000 cases of learning disorders in children and 560,000 cases of hypertension in adult males."

Asbestos is another potentially cancer-causing substance. It occurs naturally in areas that have much serpentine rock, and it can enter drinking water from asbestos-lined pipes. Thousands of these pipes installed in the 1950s have not been replaced. Asbestos particles are so small that they can't be removed by normal water treatment at municipal facilities.

Neither of these substances can be detected by sight or smell. Only special testing can identify their presence in the water we drink.

Cysts and Bacteria

In 1834, Sidney Smith wrote in a letter to Countess Gray, "He who drinks a tumbler of London water has internally in his stomach more animated beings than there are men, women and children on the face of the globe." In some ways, we have not come very far since then.

Much of our drinking water is laced with microscopic organisms, such as e-coli bacteria, giardia and cryptosporidia, which cause diarrhea and other intestinal disorders and can be deadly for people with compromised immune systems. Nearly one million people become ill from such waterborne diseases each year.

Conventional filtration by municipal water companies cannot remove these organisms completely. In 1993, an outbreak of cryptosporidia in Milwaukee, Wisconsin, infected 400,000 people, of which more than 100 died. The Center for Disease Control in Atlanta reports that "35 percent of the reported gastrointestinal illnesses among tap water drinkers each year are water-related and preventable."[6]

The Chlorine Story

By far the most devastating health hazard is chlorine, the very chemical we have used for nearly a century to make our water safe to drink.

First introduced into the U.S. public water system around 1900, chlorine quickly gained wide acceptance because it was inexpensive and effectively killed just about everything dangerous in the water (this was before the chemical pollution of the later half of the 20th century). By the 1920s, its use had spread throughout the U.S.

The results were far-reaching and spectacular. Chlorine made possible the growth of population in large cities by eliminating the health problems caused by waterborne bacteria. People no longer had to worry about periodic cholera, typhoid and dysentery epidemics.

At the time, however, almost no one gave much thought to the fact that chlorine itself was toxic. In the words of Dr. Joseph Price nearly 70 years later, "Chlorine is the greatest crippler and killer of modern times. While it prevented epidemics of one disease, it was creating another. Two decades ago, after the start of chlorinating our drinking water in 1904, the present epidemic of heart trouble, cancer and senility began."[7]

Chlorine is deadly to organic matter — that is why it is so effective against bacteria. Use chlorinated water in an aquarium and the fish will die. And what are human bodies if not organic matter? Drinking what is essentially diluted bleach can't be conducive to good health. The reason most people don't realize the consequences of chlorine is that it takes 10 to 20 years before symptoms become apparent in humans.

But scientific studies have made the dangers patently clear. Increases in heart disease, strokes, bladder and rectal cancer, premature senility, infertility and reproductive disorders have all been linked to the use of chlorine and chlorine by-products in water. According to the U.S. Council of Environmental Quality, "Cancer risk among people drinking chlorinated water is 93 percent higher than among those whose water does not contain chlorine."

In fact, chlorine is so dangerous to human beings that biologist/chemist D. Herbert Schwartz believes, "If chlorine were now proposed for the first time to be used in drinking water, it would be banned by the Food and Drug Administration."[8]

Showering

Even swimming or taking a shower in chlorinated water can be hazardous to one's health.

Many people still remember being shocked when Janet Leigh was knifed in the shower in Alfred Hitchcock's film "Psycho." The scene was so frightening at the time that for months many women refused to take a shower when alone. Little did they know that showering was dangerous indeed, but for an entirely different reason.

The human skin is like a sponge, soaking up toxic chemicals contained in water at a greater rate than can be accomplished by drinking. It also has a vastly greater surface area than the digestive system. As a result, taking a 10-minute shower can result in absorbing up to 600 percent more chlorine than drinking water all day.[9]

In addition, the water mist generated by showers spreads unhealthy chlorides, such as chloroform, throughout the house, affecting others like second-hand cigarette smoke.[10]

The Bottom Line

In continuing to use chlorine, our government has made a strategic choice to eliminate infectious diseases and offer water at a low cost to its citizens. And for good reason. Few would argue against preventing the epidemics that still ravage countries in Africa, Asia and South America.

A few U.S. cities are exploring other filtration systems to provide safe alternatives to chemical disinfectants, but the number is very small. Most municipal water companies could not afford the costly process of eliminating chlorine, even over time. The expensive pre-filters needed would drastically increase the cost of tap water to the consumer. Because only a small amount of the water delivered to homes is for drinking or bathing — more water is used to flush toilets, wash cars and water lawns during the summer — people would be unwilling to pay for it.

But the human body was never designed to become a filter for chlorine and other toxic chemicals and pollutants.

Bottled Water

More and more people are turning to bottled water. What started out as a "hip" thing for the younger crowd 20 years ago — carry a water bottle wherever you go — has become a trend. Supermarkets stock whole aisles with bottled water. Many Americans drink it regardless of the price. Evian has surpassed Perrier in sales to become the fashionable water of choice. Even the big soft drink companies have gotten into the act: Pepsi markets Aquafina and Coca Cola sells Dasani, claiming their filtration and mineral additives make them special and tastier.

Fed by media hype that would make P.T. Barnum proud, people think nothing of spending several dollars for a gallon of water (Evian, for example, costs about five dollars per gallon). But just because they believe bottled water is tastier, cleaner and healthier does not make it so.

While it may contain no chlorine, bottled water is considerably less regulated than the water that flows out of your faucet at home. Federal government oversight is practically nonexistent. There are only two requirements for bottled water — that it contain no dead organisms or visible particles. There may be minerals, bacteria and chemicals in excess of what is considered safe, and you would never know it.

The Natural Resource Defense Council (NRDC) tested over 1,000 bottles of water in 1999. In nearly a quarter of the brands, they found at least one sample with chemical contaminants at levels above accepted health limits. Consumed over a long period of time, these contaminants could cause cancer and other health problems.[11]

Bottled water sold within the state where it is manufactured does not even have to meet minimal federal standards. No wonder government and industry estimates suggest that between 25 to 30 percent of all bottled water sold in the U.S. is simply water from a local municipality — sometimes treated, sometimes not — packaged with an attractive label.

You have to read the fine print to figure out that Everest Water does not come from the snowfields of the Himalayas, but from Corpus Christi, Texas; or that Glacier Clear Water is really just tap water from Greenville, Tennessee.[12]

Another problem with bottled water, whether it comes from a spigot or a mineral spring, is that it is sold in inexpensive plastic containers, which can leach plastic compounds into the water over time. If it has been sitting on the supermarket shelf for more than 30 days, don't drink it. Some bottles have the filling date stamped on them. If they don't, check with the supermarket about when the shipment arrived. Also, check for a small triangle on the bottom of plastic bottles. The higher the number inside it, the safer the bottle (7 is optimal). The best way to store water is in glass bottles or containers made of high grade polycarbonate material.

And what about the taste? People consistently report that they prefer bottled water to tap water because it tastes better. But when the ABC News program "20/20" did a taste test using five national brands of bottled water and a sample of tap water from a drinking fountain in the middle of New York City, the tap water tied for third place with Iceland Spring (all the way from Iceland). The top contender turned out to be a discount brand from K-Mart; and dead last was the most expensive brand, the fancy French Evian water.[13]

Distilled Water

What about distilled water as an alternative?

Distilled water is produced by heating water to boiling point and then condensing the steam. This process removes most dissolved solids, such as salts, metals, minerals, asbestos fibers, and some organic chemicals, such as MTBEs and benzene. It is not effective, however, for chemicals that have a lower vaporization point than water.

Being essentially mineral-free, distilled water tends to dissolve substances it comes into contact with. The EPA has labeled it "aggressive water" because it leaches minerals, metals and others materials from whatever it passes over. As a powerful detoxification agent, distilled water can help draw poisons out of the body, helping to rid it of unwanted minerals. Some people drink it occasionally for specific health reasons, such as dissolving kidney or gall stones.

In the process, however, distilled water also removes many valuable minerals your body needs to stay healthy and in balance. Over time, as it leaches calcium and magnesium, it can cause damage to bones, teeth and tissues. The most toxic commercial beverages made from distilled water are soft drinks. Studies have consistently linked heavy consumption of soda pop (with or without sugar) to bone density loss among teenagers and a rise in bone fractures and osteoporosis.[14]

Distilled water is not a good answer to our water problems.

Water Bottles with Filters

Fortunately, there are alternatives that are healthy, tasty and cost effective — water that has been purified by filtering.

A recently developed product is the sports bottle with a filter inside. The filter is so thorough that you can convert swamp or pond water into clean, pure, good-tasting water. Portable and convenient, a filter bottle assures an ample supply of safe, purified water at a fraction of the cost of bottled water.

Water Purification Systems

Chlorine may be needed to disinfect water, but it should be removed with a good quality filter, either at the point of entry into your home or when it comes out of your kitchen or bathroom faucet. Removing all the contaminants just before use is an efficient, effective and economical solution.

There are several types of filter systems on the market, each with varying degrees of effectiveness and costs. The most popular are:

ACTIVATED CARBON FILTERS

Carbon is one of the most potent cleansing agents. One pound of carbon has a surface area equivalent to 125 acres and can absorb thousands of different chemicals and impurities.

Activated carbon has a slight electro-positive charge added to it, making it even more attractive to chemicals and impurities. As water flows through the filter bed, pollutants become attached to the surface of the carbon particles, filtering out chlorine, most organic compounds, odors and unpleasant taste.

In time, carbon filters become saturated with the chemical impurities they remove. They can also trap the bacteria found in municipal drinking water and allow them to multiply among the carbon granules. Therefore it is important to change the filter cartridge in accordance with the manufacturer's specifications.

REVERSE OSMOSIS FILTERS

In reverse osmosis units, water is forced through a semi-permeable, synthetic membrane that lets only particles of a certain size pass through. In the process, it rejects bacteria, cysts, metals — including lead and arsenic — salts, toxins and minerals. It also removes nitrates and sulphides, the by-products of fertilization most often found in agricultural areas.

While effective, this process requires a flow rate that wastes 75 percent of the tap water in the course of filtration. Like distilled water, it also has the same mineral depleting effect on the human body. If you use a reverse osmosis filter, it is highly recommended to take mineral supplements to counteract this leaching effect.

ULTRAVIOLET (UV) FILTERS
ION-EXCHANGE FILTERS
DISTILLATION FILTERS

In our view, these filters all have side effects and drawbacks that limit their usefulness as reasonable choices.

Take the Plunge

The human body was never meant to sift through the massive pollution of our times. But, as someone once said, "Either you use a filter, or you are the filter." You really owe it to yourself and to your family to have pure drinking and bathing water available at all times.

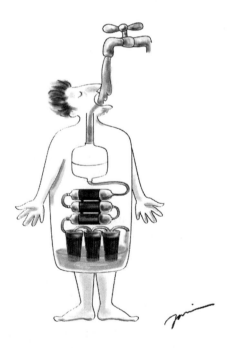

Either you use a filter, or you are the filter.

It is not difficult to obtain a high quality, cost-effective water filtration system that will allow you to enjoy pure, clean water. There are filter systems available to service part or all of your home. Most popular are units that fit on or below the kitchen counter. Easy to install shower filters can remove 99 percent of the chlorine in shower water. Whole house systems that attach at the point of entry to the house can filter all the water used for drinking, cooking, showering and bathing.

Be sure to check out documentation of what substances a filter will and will not remove. Look for a certificate from the California Department of Health, which has the most stringent requirements in the U.S., and ratings by the National Sanitation Foundation.

The Benefits of Pure Water

Water forms the basis for the saliva that keeps our mouth and throat moist. It creates the fluids that surround and cushion the joints. It regulates the body's temperature by acting as a heating and cooling system through perspiration. Water helps alleviate constipation, facilitates the absorption of food, and helps deliver vital nutrients and oxygen to all the body's cells. By removing wastes and toxins, it protects organs and tissues.

Water can raise the body's metabolism by three percent, which burns more calories and is one of the reasons that drinking water is recommended as a major part of any weight loss regimen. Nothing impacts health and well-being, and improves quality of life, like pure water.

Studies have shown that drinking plenty of water is associated with a reduction in colon, breast, bladder and kidney cancers, and decreased heart attacks and stroke.

Dehydration is one of the most common causes of daytime fatigue. An estimated 75 percent of Americans suffer from mild, chronic dehydration, much of it caused by excessive consumption of coffee and soft drinks. Many people don't realize that their headaches are the result of dehydration and could easily be cured without resorting to pain pills.

Often when we experience hunger, it is really the result of dehydration. Next time you have a craving for food that sends you to the refrigerator, drink a glass of water first and see if your desire doesn't disappear.

Make a switch to purified water and watch your health and well-being improve dramatically.

Good Water Habits

Under normal circumstances, people lose between two to three cups of water a day through perspiration and urination. But an hour of vigorous exercise can sweat out as much as a quart of water or more.

Thus, the average adult needs about eight to ten glasses of water a day. Most Americans don't come close to drinking that much. Yet many people consume more coffee or soda than that. With the way most tap water tastes, including the water served by many restaurants, it is easy to understand why people prefer flavored beverages.

With a good filter and a little determination, staying hydrated is actually easy to do.

Start and end the day with a glass of water. Since we lose water during sleep, it is a good idea to drink one glass before going to bed at night and another glass as soon as we wake up. *That's two glasses.*

Drink a glass of water about half an hour before and after lunch and dinner. Consuming it during the meal dilutes the digestive fluids in your system and makes it more difficult to digest solid food. *That's four more glasses.*

Take a sports bottle with you and sip throughout the day. That's easily *two more glasses, which totals eight!*

Do not wait to drink water until you are thirsty. By the time you feel thirsty, you may already be dehydrated. Instead, keep drinking throughout the day.

Drink an additional glass of water for each glass of coffee or alcoholic beverage. In fact, a good way to keep both hydrated and in good shape at a party is to drink a glass of water for every glass of wine or liquor.

As the American philosopher Henry David Thoreau, who understood the importance of water, said over 150 years ago, "Water is the only drink for a wise man."

In Conclusion

Exposure to chlorinated water can contribute to a host of health problems over time. Remember, either you use a filter, or you are the filter. Drinking pure, filtered water is essential to improving the quality of your life.

Having pure water is not an expensive proposition. A sports bottle, countertop kitchen filter and shower filter cost less than a dollar a day, a small price to pay for all the health and wellness benefits you will get in return.

Three Easy Steps

1. Sports bottles provide mobility and easy access throughout the day. The cost of one bottle that lasts all year is less than a meal at a good restaurant.

2. Add a countertop or below-counter filter in the kitchen for drinking and cooking. The best systems will deliver purified water at less than 10 cents a gallon. Also, invest in a shower filter. There is no point in limiting your chlorine intake orally and getting doused with it during your bath or shower.

3. Better yet, get a whole house filter that will purify all the water coming into your living quarters, and a sports bottle for drinking away from home.

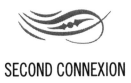

SECOND CONNEXION

Eating Right

Never eat anything you can't lift.

Miss Piggy

To say that Americans have an unhealthy relationship with food is an understatement. We consume enormous quantities of fast food, fat food and junk food. According to the World Health Organization, the average American eats 160 pounds of sugar a year. Obesity has reached near epidemic proportions. We are indeed a fat, unhealthy nation. As John Kenneth Galbraith, the American economist said, "More die in the United States from too much food than from too little."

Every few months or so, a new diet hits the market. No doubt, the latest entry in the battle of the bulge will work for a while, but fail miserably in the long run. In the words of the inimitable Jackie Gleason, "The second day of a diet is always easier than the first. By the second day, you're off it." Indeed, studies suggest that 90 percent of those who start on a new diet quit within a year and then gain an extra 10 ten pounds in the bargain.[1]

Why should this be so? Most diets cause early weight loss by restricting or eliminating the consumption of essential nutrients. They literally starve the body of what it needs. When people finally go off the diet, the body heaves a proverbial sigh of relief and stores extra fat for the next time it has to undergo deprivation. The only solution is a long-term change in lifestyle that offers a nutritionally balanced approach.

A State of Confusion

When it comes to food and eating, most people are overwhelmed by information overload. Consider the nutritional labels that were mandated in 1994 on every consumable item in the grocery store. Some people read them, many do not, and few are any wiser about how to eat well because of them. Eating guidelines disseminated by the U.S. Department of Agriculture's (USDA) have changed numerous times since the 1950s, based on recommendations by scientists. If nutritionists and scientists cannot agree, how are the rest of us going to make any sense of it?[2]

Another reason for the ongoing debate is economic self interest. The famous Food Pyramid is in its fifth edition since 1992. Many of the changes were the direct results of demands by the meat and dairy industries. The proponents of new diets often interpret information selectively and make claims to suit their purposes. No wonder people are confused. When the USDA conducted a telephone survey in 1996, it found that over 40 percent of the people interviewed agreed with the statement, "There are so many recommendations about healthy ways to eat, it's hard to know what to believe."[3]

But there is agreement among scientists and nutritionists about principles, which are unchanging. For example, the less processed and closer to the source food is, the better. There have also been recent discoveries of how the body reacts to particular foods. This chapter will discuss the basic principles that we can all agree on and use to our benefit.

Nutritional Basics

Let's begin our journey towards eating right by discussing the basics of how our body deals with food. While we may enjoy the delicious flavors and taste, the body thinks of food the way a car thinks of fuel: Does it provide the necessary energy for propulsion?

Does it offer the essential nutrients to perform the chemical reactions necessary for proper functioning?

The essential nutrients our bodies require are:

Proteins

Fats

Carbohydrates (carbs)

Vitamins

Minerals

Fiber

Water

Digestion breaks down the food we eat into simpler chemical compounds that can be absorbed through the intestinal wall and transported by the blood to the cells. There the body's metabolism converts the digested nutrients into building material or energy.

Let's look at each of these nutrients in more detail.

Proteins

After water, protein is the second most abundant substance in the human body, representing about 20 percent of its weight. Protein (from the Greek for "primary") provides the building blocks necessary for all cells to grow and to maintain their structure. During digestion, protein breaks down into amino acids that can enter the bloodstream. When the body does not receive an adequate supply of essential amino acids, it starts to break down its muscle tissue to provide energy. It also loses the means to repair damaged cells and tissue, resulting in exhaustion and greater susceptibility to illnesses.

Altogether, the body requires 22 amino acids, of which it can only produce 14. The other eight "essential amino acids" must be supplied by food. Fish, dairy, and meat products are complete protein foods, meaning that they contain all eight essential amino acids. Nuts, beans, grains and soybeans, as well as some vegetables, all are good sources of protein, but because they have only some of the eight amino acids, they need to be combined for the body to get all the protein it needs.

Fats

Unfortunately, this is one of those categories where an overabundance of terminology can be daunting and confusing. From television commercials and various news reports, you might have heard the following terms:

Fatty acids

Triglycerides

Saturated, unsaturated, mono- and polyunsaturated fat

Partially hydrogenated fat, trans fatty acids, killer fats

Essential fatty acids (EFAs), omega-3 and omega-6 fatty acids

Fats are broken down in the digestive system into **fatty acid** molecules and reassembled into **triglycerides** for transport in the bloodstream. Fats can be found in many substances, including dairy and meat products, nuts, seeds and oils. A drop of olive oil, for example, contains over a billion fatty acid molecules.

There are good fats and bad fats.

Unsaturated fats are good fats. They come in **poly-** or **mono-** forms, depending on their molecular makeup. Vegetable oils are the best examples of unsaturated fats. **Mono-unsaturated** fats, such as those found in olive and canola oil, can even lower cholesterol.

Saturated fats are found in meat and dairy products, such as milk and cheese. The body needs some of these fats, but a diet high in saturated fats tends to clog arteries and is considered unhealthy.

Partially hydrogenated fat and **trans fatty acids**, produced by heating polyunsaturated oil, are used in many packaged snacks, cookies and fried foods. Also known as **killer fats**, they are now considered extremely harmful. Since our bodies are incapable of eliminating them, they build up and cause depressed immune functions, raised cholesterol and increased susceptibility to degenerative diseases.[4]

There are **essential fatty acids (EFAs)**, however, and by limiting our intake of fat in general, we may end up depriving our bodies of the fats we need to survive. The most familiar EFAs are **omega-3** and **omega-6** fatty acids, which have been shown to speed up the healing of wounds and improve the condition of skin and hair. They also play a role in immune functions and may help reduce the occurrence of degenerative diseases and cancers.[5]

The best food sources of omega-6 fats are pumpkin and sunflower seeds, walnuts and almonds. Omega-3 fats are most prominent in flax seeds and fatty fish, such as mackerel, herring, sardines, trout and salmon. Both omega-3 and omega-6 fatty acids are also available as nutritional supplements (discussed in a later chapter).

Fats can be divided into two categories:

1. Beneficial fats, such as unsaturated fats and EFAs.

2. Harmful fats, such as partially hydrogenated fats and trans fatty acids.

To optimize health, it makes sense to eat more essential fats and to avoid harmful ones as much as possible. As the old English proverb advises, "Don't dig your grave with your own knife and fork."

Carbohydrates

Carbohydrates are the energy workhorses of the body. Powering muscles and aiding in the digestion and assimilation of all foods, carbohydrates — or carbs — provide the energy our bodies need to survive.

Foods containing starches and sugars are the source of carbohydrates. Simple sugars, such as glucose, fructose (in fruits), lactose (in milk) and sucrose (white sugar or "table sugar") are absorbed by the body without having to be broken down by the digestive process. If you drink a solution of water and glucose, for example, the glucose passes directly from your intestines into the bloodstream.

Starches, found in whole grains and vegetables, are also known as complex carbohydrates. Because it takes time for enzymes to break them down into glucose molecules before they can be assimilated into the bloodstream, these carbohydrates are absorbed more slowly. The sugar from a can of soda enters the bloodstream at a rate of about 30 calories per minute. A complex carbohydrate does so at two calories a minute.[6]

When you eat a candy bar or drink a can of soda, the glucose level in the blood rises quickly. In response, the pancreas secretes a large quantity of insulin to keep blood glucose levels from rising too high. The body needs insulin to survive because too much glucose in the blood is toxic for the brain. Such a radical insulin response results in blood sugar falling to levels that are too low. This in turn leads to an adrenalin surge, which can cause nervousness and irritability, often followed by eating more simple carbs in an effort to raise the blood sugar quickly.

This spike and collapse in insulin levels is a self-replicating cycle that dramatically affects our moods and our sense of alertness and well-being. When people "crash" on the downward side, they crave food like an addict wanting a fix, compounding the situation by eating more sweets and simple carbs. Over time, this process increases our body's resistance to insulin, leading to high insulin levels, poor sugar metabolism, and type II diabetes.

This glycemic cycle also contributes to obesity, because the body releases no stored fat during the insulin secreting stage. Instead, it deposits any excess sugar in fat cells, which have a virtually unlimited capacity and can swell to 1,000 times their original size!

When we eat complex carbs or a balanced meal, this roller-coaster ride of glucose and hormone levels does not happen, because glucose absorption is much slower.

THE GLYCEMIC INDEX

The glycemic index measures the rapid surges and declines in blood sugar and insulin levels, which lead to adrenalin rushes and cravings for even more carbs.

It turns out that there are certain foods that cause a rapid release of insulin, which results in the rollercoaster described above. Many researchers now believe that this cycle of binging and craving underlies today's epidemics of obesity and cardiovascular disease.[7]

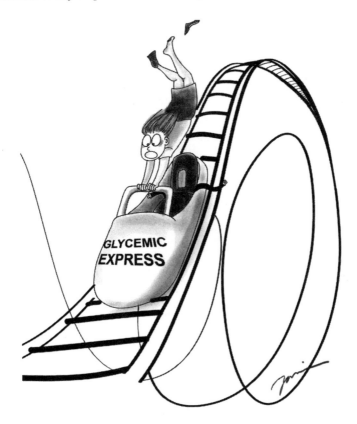

Whooooooaaaahhhh!

Not surprisingly, highly refined foods, such as corn flakes, instant rice and bread, as well as sweet fruit like papayas and raisins, rank high on the glycemic index. In the low to middle ranges are pastas, pumpernickel bread, oranges, apples, cherries, kidney beans, lentils, peas, yogurt, peanuts and soy beans.

Low Glycemic Foods: 1-60

Dairy
Whole Milk (30)
Yogurt, fruit (36)
Yogurt, plain (14)

Fruit
Apple (38)
Banana (56)
Cherries (22)
Grapefruit (25)
Orange (43)
Peach (42)
Pear (58)
Plum (55)

Vegetables
Corn, Sweet (56)
Carrots (49)
Peas (48)
Potato, sweet (54)
Potato, white (56)

Legumes
All beans are below 60
Soy beans are the lowest (16)

Cereal Grains
Basmati white rice (58)
Bulgur wheat (48)
Oatmeal, old-fashioned (48)

Soup
Tomato Soup (54)
Lentil Soup (63)

Other
Apple Cinnamon muffin (44
Blueberry muffin (59)
Pasta (32-46)
Popcorn (55)
Orange juice (46)

High Glycemic FOODS: 60-120

Ice Cream (87)

Watermelon (72)
Cantaloupe (65)
Pineapple (66)
Raisins (64)

Beets (64)
Yams (71)
Parsnips (97))
Pumpkin (107)

Millet (71)
Cornmeal (68)
Commercial cereals (65-85)

Split Pea Soup (66)

Bagel, plain (72)
Doughnut (76)
French fries (75)
Pretzels (83)
Gatorade (78)

We recommend eating complex and unrefined carbohydrates that have a low to moderate glycemic index, or combining high with low glycemic foods (as in a smoothie), so you can get benefit of fruit and colorful vegetables without negative effects.

Vitamins and Minerals

We will discuss vitamins and minerals in greater detail in the chapter on supplementation. For now let us just say that vitamins and minerals work in combination with enzymes to ensure that the nutrients of foods are properly used for cellular maintenance, energy, and support of the body's immune system.

Fiber

Not everything we eat can be digested. Fiber is the umbrella name we give to that part of food which our bodies cannot absorb. Fiber passes through unaffected by our digestive system. While it doesn't provide nourishment, it does slow down the digestive process by adding bulk, and acts as a cleansing agent for the digestive tract. Fiber-rich food also tends to have a lower glycemic index.

The fiber we eat on a regular basis comes in the form of cellulose, hemicellulose or pectin. **Pectin** is found mostly in fruits. **Hemicellulose** is found in the hulls of grains, such as wheat. Bran, for example, is hemicellulose. **Cellulose** is found in the skin of fruit and vegetables.

Water and Other Liquids

We have already discussed the importance of pure, filtered water to health and wellness. Let's look at some of the other liquids many people consume during the day.

Sodas: It will come as no surprise that we are not fans of soda of any kind. The sugar content and high acidity in regular sodas are simply unhealthy, an invitation to climb on the insulin-glucose roller-coaster. In addition, the phosphoric acid and distilled water in both regular and diet sodas are now considered a likely cause of bone density loss.[8]

Alcohol: We recommend keeping alcohol consumption to a minimum. Alcohol converts to sugar quickly and has a high glycemic index. There is, however, some research that suggests one glass of red wine a day may be beneficial to health because it contains antioxidants. If you choose to drink, use moderation and follow up each alcoholic beverage with a glass of water.

Milk: Despite the claims of the dairy industry, milk may not be good for you. It is loaded with fat (even low fat and skim milk), most of it saturated and hard to digest. Studies suggest that, rather than providing the essential calcium we need, milk actually leaches it from the bones, contributing to osteoporosis. Many adults are lactose intolerant, developing rashes, headaches and irritability from consuming milk. Add to that the concentration of growth hormones and antibiotics that cows are injected with, and it is better to avoid milk and dairy products altogether.[9] Use alternatives like soy milk and olive oil whenever possible, and you will feel better and become healthier.

That completes our tour through the essential nutrients and foods that our bodies need. We now turn to how the energy from food is measured.

Calories

Calories have been the rage for years. People are counting them, cutting them, and scouring the labels on food packages in supermarkets for them. As you may remember from high school chemistry, a calorie — the name comes from Latin for "heat" — is a unit of energy. We have come to associate them with food, but calories apply to anything that contains energy. For example, a can of regular soda contains 200 calories, while a gallon of gasoline contains roughly 31,000 calories.

Our bodies "burn" the calories in food through the metabolic process by which enzymes break down food into glucose, fatty acids and amino acids. These are transported to all the cells, where they react with oxygen to release their stored energy. In terms of energy output:

1 gram of carbohydrates = 4 calories

1 gram of protein = 4 calories

1 gram of fat = 9 calories

The average human body needs 1,800 to 2,000 calories a day just to function, depending on height, weight, gender, age and activity levels. Keeping the heart beating, the lungs breathing, the kidneys functioning, and the body temperature stabilized accounts for two-thirds of all calories burned. Physical activity, such as getting out of bed, walking, lifting, bending and just generally moving around is the next largest calorie burner. The digestive process — it takes energy to break down food to its basic elements — takes about 10 percent.

If you take in fewer or more calories than your body burns, you will lose or gain fat, respectively. Your body will store 3,500 extra calories as one pound of fat. If you burn 3,500 more calories than you need over time, by exercising or eating less, your body will convert one pound of stored fat into energy to make up for the deficit.

Not All Calories Are Alike

In a 1956 study, four groups of people were fed 1,000 calories per day for 10 days. The people in Group 1 received 90 percent of their calories from fat. Group 2 got 90 percent of its calories from protein. Group 3 obtained 42 percent of its calories from carbohydrates, 29 percent from protein, and 29 percent from fat. And Group 4 got 90 percent from carbs. The results over the course of the testing period were very interesting:

Group 1 (90 percent fat) lost 1.01 pounds per day

Group 2 (90 percent protein) lost 0.8 pounds per day

Group 3 (42/29/29) lost 1.01 pounds per day

Group 4 (90 percent carbs) gained 0.1 pounds per day

Note that the highest weight loss came about from the group eating 42 percent carbohydrates, 29 percent protein and 29 percent fat. (Although Group 1 lost the same amount of weight, it is not worth considering, since existing on fat alone is a regimen guaranteed to shorten anyone's life.) Round off the figures, and you get a proportion of 40/30/30 for carbs/protein/fat, a healthy, balanced approach. Of course, this assumes eating a diet of complex, unrefined carbohydrates and healthy fats.

No one knows if there is an ideal diet. After all, people have different metabolisms. Not everyone responds negatively to high glycemic food. It is also important to remember that eating well represents only one aspect of wellness. But there seems to be one cuisine, developed over centuries, that includes most of the discoveries we have made about healthy eating; namely, the diet used by most Mediterranean people — Spanish, Italian, Greek, etc.

The Mediterranean diet is high in complex carbohydrates, which have a low glycemic index and are high in fiber, fruit and vegetables. It also includes cheese, eggs, fish, fowl, garlic, onions and yogurt. Red meat is eaten only in small quantities. Wine is consumed in moderation, mostly during meals. Hard liquor is not part of the menu. According to the New England Journal of Medicine, people who eat a Mediterranean-style diet have a 25 percent reduced risk of dying from cancer or heart disease.

Surprisingly, the Mediterranean diet contains a greater amount of fat than recommended by many American health practitioners, but it is mostly "good" fat, found in nuts, avocados, fish and olive oil. Fats do not trigger insulin release the way the metabolism of carbohydrates does. Despite its high fat content, the Mediterranean diet is good for the heart.[10]

Overall, the Mediterranean diet naturally follows the 40/30/30 ratio of carbs to proteins to fat. Above all, it has great variety and is delicious, a pleasure to the palate. Since it is as much a cuisine as a diet, it is fully integrated into the lifestyle of the people that consume it. There is nothing fast food about it. Its practitioners also tend to eat smaller portions and take their time to appreciate meals in the company of others.

A Handful of Suggestions

Here are some general principles of eating well we can all agree on:

EAT MORE SLOWLY

Digestion starts with chewing. In the words of Charles T. Copeland, "To eat is human, to digest divine." Our grandparents were right when they exhorted us to chew well and slowly. Most people don't chew enough, depriving themselves of the first enzyme to start the process of breaking down food — saliva. This prevents the stomach enzymes from doing their job well. The larger pieces of food sit there, undigested, rotting, causing bloating and indigestion.

A good rule to follow instead is: If it's chunky, don't swallow it. Keep chewing.

Another benefit of eating slowly is that the brain catches on that its hunger pangs are being satisfied. It takes 20 minutes before the brain registers that nourishment is being consumed. People who eat on the run don't have time for that message to reach their brains. As a result, they eat more than necessary and short circuit their digestive process, causing bloating and heartburn. If you are going to eat on the run, it is better not to eat at all.

Above all, eating slowly allows you to appreciate the meal, the tastes, the smells, the delights. In France, Italy, Russia and Germany, people frequently sit down to meals that take several hours.

SMALLER PORTIONS

When people are diagnosed with diabetes, they often pay the first visit of their lives to a nutritionist. One of the things they learn, usually to their surprise, is what a portion of rice or chicken or broccoli actually looks like. Invariably, it is much smaller than what they are used to piling on their plates.

Eating smaller portions makes an enormous difference to one's waistline. Author Rita Mae Brown suggests that the best way to lose weight is to pile everything one normally eats on a plate, and then take a knife and remove half.[11]

Another way of measuring proper portions is to use your hand. The portion of protein consumption in a meal — especially meats and fish — should be no larger than the palm of your hand (or a deck of playing cards). You can divide carbs into healthy and unhealthy. For the healthy kind — moderate to low glycemic, unrefined, such as fruit, vegetables, whole grains — you can have two fists worth. For the unhealthy kind — high glycemic, refined, such as bread, pasta and other starches — you should never have more than one fist, if any at all. This is a good way to follow the 40/30/30 rule.

EAT FIVE TIMES A DAY

Studies suggest that eating smaller quantities of food more frequently reduces the feeling of hunger which leads to binging and smoothes out the insulin spike and collapse cycle.

Never let more than five hours pass without a meal or snack, except at night. If you eat before going to bed, some of the food will not be metabolized while you sleep. Instead, it will get stored as fat.

EAT GOOD QUALITY FOOD

As an anonymous writer quipped, "Your stomach shouldn't be a waist basket." Eat less processed, less treated and less refined food. When it comes to fruits and vegetables, the fresher and less cooked the better. As for meat, eat lean rather than fat, and organic if you can get it (to avoid added hormones and antibiotics).

SLOW DOWN AND ENJOY YOUR FOOD

Eating right means taking the time to enjoy the food you eat. As novelist Virginia Woolf said, "One cannot think well, love well, sleep well, if one has not dined well."

A Few Helpful Hints

- Don't go to the supermarket when you are hungry.

- Eat only half of restaurant meals. Take the other half home for lunch the next day.

- Substitute yogurt, fresh fruit or nuts for chips, candy and other junk-food snacks.

- If you do all the right things 90 percent of the time, it is okay to indulge your cravings the other 10 percent.

Wellness Is a Journey

Make consistent small changes. For some that may be weaning themselves off soda; for others it may be deliberately introducing one more vegetable per meal. Stick with it when you have setbacks — they are a normal part of the process. And celebrate when you reach a milestone — like a month without extra sugar.

It may seem complicated at first, but a small investment of time to develop a healthy eating program will pay vast dividends. You will feel better, find more joy in eating and be well on the way to improving your health and your prospects for growing older with fewer health problems.

Remember, eating well is a lifelong pursuit. As Cicero, the Roman orator said over 2,000 years ago, "You should eat to live, not live to eat." The benefits of being thinner and healthier outweigh any personal sacrifice you may have to make.

Three Easy Steps

1. For carbohydrates: Avoid simple sugars and refined carbs in favor of complex, unrefined carbs. Eat more fruit and vegetables.

2. For protein: Limit your meat intake. Get more protein from beans, grains and vegetables. Choose leaner, lower fat sources of protein, such as chicken, fish, or lean cuts of meat.

3. For fats: Avoid saturated and hydrogenated trans fatty acids. Use cold pressed olive and canola oil instead. Be sure to get omega-3 and omega-6 from nuts, seeds, avocados and fish or via nutritional supplements.

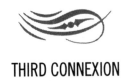

THIRD CONNEXION

ELIMINATING TOXINS

*There is so much pollution in the air now that if it weren't
for our lungs there'd be no place to put it all.*

ROBERT ORBEN, AMERICAN HUMORIST

In 1912, Dr. Alexis Carrel, a Nobel Prize winning scientist, began
a remarkable experiment. Under his direction, researchers at
the Rockefeller Institute in New York took a small piece from the
heart of a chicken embryo and placed it in a laboratory flask. By
supplying it with nutrients and water and removing the waste it
produced, they succeeded in keeping it alive and growing for 34
years. Quite an accomplishment, considering that the normal life
span of a chicken is only 10 years. What is even more amazing is
that the researchers stopped the experiment because they became
convinced that they could keep the chicken cells alive forever.

The outcome suggests that the well-being of organic, living cells
depends on receiving proper nourishment and being able to
eliminate the toxins that build up in the normal course of existence.
The implications for human beings, whose bodies are made
up entirely of organic cells, are profound. Since we completely
regenerate every single cell in our bodies over the course of seven
years, we can potentially affect our health, well-being and even the
aging process by what we consume and how we get rid of waste.

There is a great deal of information about the role of food and water in promoting a healthy lifestyle, which was addressed in the previous chapters. Less well understood is the importance of elimination or detoxification, which is as critical to our well-being as the air we breathe.

Detoxification is a Natural Process

The human body has a number of systems to cleanse itself. It expels wastes and toxins through the bowels, filters them through the liver and kidneys, exudes them through the skin, and exhales them via the lungs. Stool, urine, sweat and breath are all part of the body's self-cleansing mechanisms.

The path to good health is straightforward. Choose wisely what you put into your body and make sure that your elimination systems work at maximum capacity.

Unfortunately, it is not that simple.

Our Toxic Environment

Toxins have always been around us. But over the past 100 years, we have created a host of chemicals that never existed before. In the process, we have saturated our environment with toxic waste and products hazardous to our health.

Our air is polluted with lead emitted by automobiles. Dioxins and PCBs issue from the smokestacks of factories where plastic products are manufactured. Benzene, known to cause leukemia, comes from car exhaust fumes, gasoline, plastics and cleansers. In a study that analyzed the breath of 235 New Jersey residents, 89 percent had traces of benzene.[1]

Our drinking water is laced with pesticides, fertilizers, organo-phosphates and heavy metals. Our food is packed with hormones, preservatives, artificial coloring and sweeteners. You would not spray a can of bug killer into your mouth, yet when you eat unwashed fruit and vegetables, you ingest the same pesticides — all linked to various debilitating diseases.

Even our homes are no longer safe. From fluoro-carbons in carpeting to cleaning products and killer pesticides in the hall closet or under the kitchen counter, we are surrounded by toxic chemicals. Many commercial shampoos, deodorants, hair dyes, cosmetics and fragrances contain ingredients such as aluminum, formaldehyde, coal tar and phthalates (plastic compounds) that have been linked to cancer and birth defects.[2]

We absorb mercury from the air, from our dental fillings and from polluted fish. We take in phthalates that leach from plastic wrapping into the meat and vegetables we eat. An EPA study found that 100 percent of human fat samples contained styrene, which can cause cancer or other health disorders. Styrene is all-pervasive, emitted as gas from our computers and found in numerous everyday plastic products, such as plastic bottles and Styrofoam cups.[3]

In Western countries, we use more than 75,000 chemicals and develop over 1,000 new ones each year! Even a chemical like DDT, banned in the U.S. decades ago because it is such a powerful carcinogen, continues to show up in our water supply and food. From there it makes its way into our bodies and takes its toll on our health. And we still manufacture it and sell it to Third World countries.[4]

Indeed, pollution has spread to every corner of the globe. Climb Mt. Everest and you will breathe dioxins and PCBs when you get to the top. Go back to nature and you will find, as scientists have, man-made chemicals in pristine lakes and rivers, and among plants and wildlife in remote areas accessible only by hiking or helicopters.

We are living in the equivalent of a chemical laboratory, a highly toxic environment from which there is no escape; and the consequences for our health and well-being are devastating.

Since the advent of man-made chemical pollutants, there has been an unprecedented rise in chronic diseases such as Parkinson's and Alzheimer's, auto-immune diseases such as lupus, and all kinds of cancer. Depression has been on the rise as well. Chemical pollution is the likely candidate as the cause of all these ills.[5] According to the Columbia University School of Public Health, 95 percent of all cancer is caused by diet and the environment.

Hormones and chemicals that mimic hormones in the body confuse the endocrine system, leading to premature breast development and an early onset of puberty in young girls, as well as breast cancer in adult women and prostate cancer in men. At the same time, sperm count and fertility rates have dropped throughout the industrialized West. More and more babies are born prematurely. Again, the rise of chemical toxins in our environment is a leading suspect.[6]

Old-time Detoxification in the Modern Chemical Lab

The human body was never designed to cope with the assault of chemical pollution faced by many Americans. It is simply overwhelmed by the variety and quantity of toxins, unable to eliminate them in the normal course of detoxification. In time, they devastate the immune system, metabolic functions, and physical and emotional health. They literally kill us.

Just how dangerous these chemical pollutants are to human beings is demonstrated when people are exposed to excessive quantities. One of the earliest examples was the mercury poisoning of Minamata Bay in Japan by a petrochemical company. The families of the local fishermen ate large quantities of the contaminated fish. Later, people started to show a variety of alarming symptoms — numbness in limbs and lips, slurred speech, incoherent shouting and brain damage. Babies were stillborn or suffered serious birth defects. Over 3,000 people have been diagnosed with "Minamata Disease."

The movie "Erin Brokovich" was based on an actual case in which the Pacific Gas & Electric Company of California polluted a community's ground water with hexavalent chromium, a deadly carcinogen that especially affects the lungs. In 1973, the residents of Love Canal, near Niagara Falls, New York, had to be evacuated when it was discovered that their community had been built on a landfill that covered a chemical dumping ground. Residents suffered from cancer and respiratory problems, and their children experienced frequent illnesses.

There are numerous such "hot zones" in the U.S., the legacy of years of toxic waste dumping by chemical companies. According to Phil Clapp, President of National Environmental Trust, "One in six Americans lives within a mile of a major toxic waste site." The EPA has a "superfund" to help clean up the most serious cases, but it is woefully inadequate to deal with the problem.

Stockpiling and Compounding the Problem

Most of us are fortunate not to live in such dire circumstances. But we take in toxic substances in smaller amounts. The EPA and chemical and food industries claim that the trace quantities we consume are harmless. What they neglect to mention is that because the body is unable to eliminate what we inhale and ingest, toxins build up over time, leading to severe health consequences.

It may take 15 to 20 years before the cumulative effects show up and symptoms emerge. According to René Dubos, the French-American bacteriologist, "The most pathological effects of pollution are extremely delayed and indirect." When they appear, many of us don't make the connection. We blame auto-immune disorders and degenerative diseases on growing old.[7] And because individuals respond differently, many doctors don't recognize the symptoms for what they really are. They prescribe drugs, which may or may not help, but never get to the root cause.[8]

Around the turn of the century, for example, detectives and forensic scientists inhaled excessive quantities of mercury from the powder used to dust for fingerprints. But it was not until the 1940s that doctors made the connection between the array of symptoms — excessive salivation, stomach pains, insomnia, tremors and irritability — and the real cause: chronic mercury poisoning.[9]

In some cases, small amounts can be as harmful as large-scale exposure. Independent research scientists are discovering how small doses of pesticides, especially during critical periods of fetal development and childhood, can have serious, long-term effects. We have known for some time of the dangers of lead exposure and its devastating effect on the brain development of children. Over the past 30 years, there has been an increase of diseases such as asthma, autism and attention deficit disorders, childhood brain cancer and leukemia. Although scientists do not have a full explanation for these increases, early exposure to environmental toxins is a leading candidate.[10]

There is even chemical pollution in the womb these days. A recent study that tested blood samples of umbilical cords of healthy newborn babies discovered that they had an average of 200 contaminants in their blood. Among them were 76 known carcinogens, 79 chemicals known to cause birth defects, and 94 substances toxic to the nervous system and the brain. They also included industrial lubricants and pesticides that have been banned in the U.S. for decades.[11]

In the face of these alarming developments, perhaps most troubling of all is that no one seems to be minding the chemical supply closet. In July, 2005, the U.S. Government Accountability Office released a report criticizing the EPA for poor oversight. According to the report, "The EPA does not routinely assess existing chemicals, has limited information on their health and environmental risks, and has issued few regulations controlling such chemicals."

These are life and death matters, yet few people pay attention.

Reversing the Trend

We are a far cry from the optimal environment that made Dr. Carrel's chicken cells virtually immortal. In fact, the problem of toxic waste in our system is so pervasive that some researchers have referred to our bodies, which consist of about 70 percent water, as a toxic chemical soup.

But there is hope. Even with long-term exposure, we can decrease our toxicity and improve our chances for a longer, healthier life.

That is why cleansing above and beyond the body's own resources is a must, and why it is so important to make detoxification a regular part of your journey to wellness. While it may not be possible to completely eliminate all toxins from our bodies, it is well within our power to make smart choices that significantly affect our health and well-being.

We recommend addressing the need for detoxification in three stages:

1. Decrease sources of toxicity.

2. Improve the body's own elimination process.

3. Remove toxins already stored inside you.

Decrease Sources of Toxicity

We take substances into our body through our mouth, our lungs and our skin. The fewer pollutants we absorb, the better. Many people spend the majority of their waking and sleeping hours at home. Thus, the home is as good a place as any to start the process of decontamination. Many toxic chemicals can be eliminated simply by making more deliberate choices in the supermarket.[12]

AT HOME

Take a tour of your house with fresh eyes. What can you eliminate, what can you change?

The average carpet releases more than a dozen chemicals in gas form, from fluoro-carbons to formaldehyde, benzene and styrene. Anderson Labs took a small patch of carpet that customers had been complaining about and placed it on the bottom of a glass jar with some mice. The next morning the mice were dead. There are carpets available now that limit chemicals. Wood and tile floors make good alternatives.

Consider non-chemical cleaning agents and insecticides. Try lemon juice for ants and citronella plants and candles for mosquitoes. Use pesticides only as a last resort. Before using heavy chemical household cleaners and disinfectants, try soap and water first.

Most people don't think about the fire retardants in their mattresses and pillows, or paints, solvents, oils, grease and lawn mower gas cans in their basement or garage — all of them containing hazardous pollutants.

Molds can set off hormonal changes in the body, trigger allergy symptoms and cause cancer. If possible, install a fresh air circulation system and filter as part of your air conditioner to remove dust and other particulates from the air,

Avoid artificial fragrances and air fresheners. Limit the number of synthetic cosmetics and personal care products — cleansers, deodorants and conditioners. They can contain harmful unregulated chemicals. We recommend using natural alternatives instead.

PURE WATER

We have already discussed the necessity of pure water. You do not need to be the filter for all the metals, chemicals, bacteria and spores coming out of your tap. At the very least, install good filters in your home and let them do the job for you.

THE FOOD YOU EAT

Food is often overlooked as a source of toxicity, but it can contain many pesticides. In the words of Dr. Jay Kenny, a nutrition research specialist, "Most people dig their grave with their teeth, but you have to eat badly for decades before it starts to show damage."13

Pesticides are powerful chemicals, designed to kill bugs, weeds, fungi and vermin. Claims by pesticide manufacturers and the government that "there is no conclusive evidence of harm to humans" are misleading. After all, the EPA asserted that highly toxic pesticides like DDT and chlordane were safe, up to the day that it banned them!

Apples, for example, are sprayed as often as 14 times a season. Animal grain and feed is grown with pesticides and herbicides, and they become part of our food chain.

Based on studies, the Environmental Working Group (EWG) and Stonyfield Farm published a list of "The Dirty Dozen," the 12 most contaminated fruits and vegetables, which all contain multiple pesticides.[14] Here it is, along with a list of the 12 least contaminated produce items:

12 Most contaminated	12 Least Contaminated
Apples	Asparagus
Bell Peppers	Avocados
Celery	Bananas
Cherries	Broccoli
Imported Grapes	Cauliflower
Nectarines	Corn (sweet)
Peaches	Kiwi
Pears	Mangoes
Potatoes	Onions
Red raspberries	Papaya
Spinach	Pineapples
Strawberries	Peas (sweet)

EWG recommends buying "The Dirty Dozen," in organic form. We suggest buying only organic produce, if possible. Why eat any pesticides if you can avoid them?

A FEW OTHER EATING TIPS

- Eat fewer processed foods, which usually contain chemical additives.

- Don't microwave food in plastic containers, which will leach phthalates. Use glass or ceramic containers instead.

- Eat less meat and avoid high-fat dairy products, which contain higher levels of some pollutants.

- Avoid seafood known to contain high quantities of PCBs and mercury. Eat wild Alaskan salmon and canned salmon instead.

Start with the things you can fix with relatively little effort. It is probably easier to change your eating habits than to redo the flooring in your house or to install a state-of-the-art air circulation system. Remember, every step you take helps in your journey toward well-being. As Dr. Andrew Weil advises, "The best way to detoxify is to stop putting toxic things into the body and depend upon its own mechanism (to cleanse itself)."

Improve the Body's Own Elimination Process

Toxins tend to concentrate in the liver and gastrointestinal tract, the two major systems responsible for eliminating toxins from the body. According to Dr. Richard Schulze, "The first step in everyone's health program should be stimulating, cleaning and toning all the elimination organs, and the bowel is the best place to begin."

THE BOWELS

Keeping the bowels clean and active is key. Constipation is more common than in previous eras because we are less active than our ancestors. We eat processed food that does not include enough roughage, we do not drink enough water, and we spend hours each day sitting. As a result, many toxins stay in the bowels longer than they should and in some cases become reabsorbed.

A change in diet is a good first step. Eat more fruit, vegetables, whole grains and other foods high in fiber. Hydrate regularly — drink 8-10 glasses of water a day. Any exercise that shakes up your body, such as walking, running, dancing or jumping, is helpful. You should have at least one bowel movement a day, preferably two to three.

IMPROVE LIVER FUNCTION

The liver is the second largest organ in the body after the skin. It is involved with virtually all of the biochemical processes necessary to grow, fight disease, supply nutrients, provide energy and aid in reproduction. Since the liver receives close to 90 percent of the blood that comes from the stomach and the intestines, one of its primary jobs is to remove toxins. It converts them into small, marble-like packets that it dumps via the gall bladder into the bowels, from where they are excreted.

When the liver gets stressed by excess waste or is unable to eliminate pollutants, the body suffers. When the problem becomes chronic, all kinds of health problems can occur.

The easiest way to strengthen the liver is through a healthy diet, avoiding alcohol, drugs, saturated fats and trans fatty acids. Garlic, ginger, citrus juice and olive oil can be used as a natural liver flush. There are also many nutritional supplements available to support healthy liver function, including alpha-lipoic acid, milk thistle and dandelion root.

COMBATING FREE RADICALS

Free radicals weaken the walls of cells and upset the body's metabolism, creating extra toxic products. These poisonous wastes interfere with inter-cell communication, upset DNA and protein synthesis, decrease energy, and generally hamper important chemical processes. In time, they lead to premature aging and diseases such as cancer.

Free radicals are created by chemical toxins, heavy metals, drugs (including alcohol and tobacco), radiation and strenuous exercise. One of the most powerful producers of free radicals is oxygen. In the same way that an apple cut in half turns brown due to the interaction with oxygen in the air, or that iron corrodes over time, our bodies "rust" and age faster when oxygen-generated free radicals have their way.

Fortunately, there is an antidote — antioxidants — which bind free radicals, rendering them harmless. A variety of antioxidants, such as beta-carotene and vitamins C and E, can be found in foods like carrots and broccoli. Maximum advantage can be obtained by taking antioxidant supplements in addition to eating a healthful, balanced diet.

Remove Toxins Already Stored Inside You

One of the ways the body copes with toxins it cannot eliminate
— heavy metals and phthalates, for example — is to store them in
fat tissues. As cells grow and regenerate, they include these toxins,
stockpiling them over time. In the process, they lodge throughout
the body, in organs and in the brain, where they interfere with
metabolism, damage cells, drain the body of energy and make
it more susceptible to diseases. Heart disease, cancer, diabetes,
arthritis and fatigue syndromes are all linked to the accumulation
of poisonous chemicals in the body.[14]

Fortunately, it is possible to get rid of them, to detoxify or cleanse
them from your system.

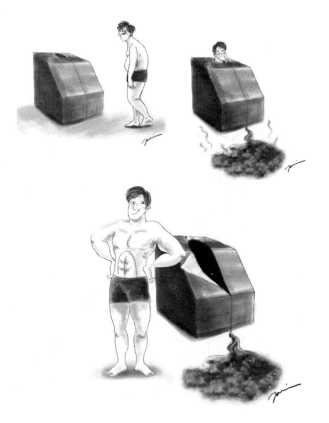

Detoxification can make you feel like a new man.

Connie came to Dr. Watts two years ago. She had been trying to lose weight without success and was in despair. She felt that unless she did, she would not be able to improve her health. Suspecting that toxins were deposited in her fat cells, Dr. Watts asked if she got sick when she started to lose weight. That turned out to be the case: every time Connie went on a weight loss program, like clockwork she became sick within 10 to 14 days. A urine test revealed that she had above normal levels of lead, antimony and gadolinium. Once she underwent detoxification, the weight began to slowly come off without ill effect.

JUICE FASTING

One helpful practice is to do a juice cleanse once a month. Give your gastrointestinal system a rest by spending a day without solid food, sipping herbal teas, water and fruit and vegetable juices.

COLONICS

Although many people are uncomfortable with the idea, many health practitioners recommend colonic irrigation to support cleansing of the large bowel. Colonics use filtered, purified water to flush out accumulated bowel encrustation, and should be administered by a licensed professional. Because the process also washes out enzymes and bacteria necessary for good digestion, it is important to replenish them afterwards by eating yogurt or taking probiotic supplements.

CHELATION

Long accepted as a method of detoxifying the body of heavy metals, such as mercury and lead, chelation therapy has become a treatment popular with many doctors of integrative and holistic medicine. Chelating agents can be taken orally or intravenously. In the later case, they must be administered under the supervision of a qualified healthcare practitioner. Since the process removes many essential nutrients along with toxic elements, it is important to replace them with vitamin and mineral supplements, as described in Chapter 4.

SAUNAS

By far the most powerful and effective way of detoxifying the body is by using a sauna. Invented by Finns over 2,000 years ago, saunas generate dry heat with heated rocks, which forces the body to sweat profusely, causing it to eliminate chemical, metal and other toxins through the skin. It is interesting to note that the tradition of sweat lodges for physical and spiritual cleansing was first practiced in this country by Native Americans.

For people who find the Finnish version of saunas hard on their lungs and eyes, there is a good modern alternative — far-infrared saunas, which generate radiant heat similar to the invisible spectrum of sunlight. They are more efficient, producing the same intense sweating and detoxification at lower temperatures and in shorter time periods.

Obviously, a sauna represents a considerable financial investment — home models can be purchased for a few thousand dollars. But the results are very much worth the investment.

MERCURY DENTAL FILLINGS

The subject of amalgamated mercury dental fillings is controversial. Despite having been used for 200 years, during the 1990s questions were raised about their safety because of their high mercury content. Although there are no confirmed studies to back up suggestions that they leak mercury into the body, there is considerable anecdotal evidence that some people develop multiple sclerosis and arthritic conditions because of low level mercury poisoning from dental fillings.[15] If you suspect that you are suffering from such mercury poisoning, have yourself tested. If you have high levels, you can have the fillings replaced and use chelation to remove the accumulated mercury from your system.

The Stress of Detoxifying

We have discussed the way toxins stress the immune system, damage cells, and upset hormone and enzyme systems in the body. Additional stress occurs when the body works to detoxify, because it uses up valuable energy and nutrients in the process. Every time we eliminate chemicals we absorb from the environment, we use up an important detox nutrient called glutathione. Created by the body from three amino acids, it can neutralize literally hundreds of environmental chemicals and pull them out of the blood, into the liver and then into the bowels for excretion.

But the depletion will leave the body vulnerable to the next exposure to toxins. The only way to counter the problem is to eat healthy food that provides nourishment for the body to make new detoxifiers like glutathione. A body fed primarily on junk food doesn't stand a chance in the battle against toxic chemicals.

In extreme cases, toxins are released faster than the body can eliminate them, producing disease-like symptoms such as headaches, nausea, vomiting and skin rashes. In general, the more toxins there are to eliminate, the "sicker" one gets as they come out.

It is important to remember that such responses are a necessary part of the healing and cleansing process, and will only last a relatively short time. If you are experiencing such reactions, back off the program and proceed more slowly, unless you are on a major detoxing program being supervised by a physician.

For this reason, we recommend that any radical detoxing program — colonics, chelation, extended diets, or herbal treatments — be performed under the supervision of a licensed professional or a medical doctor.

When you have regained your health, make detoxification a regular part of your life. Remember René Dubos' mantra of hope, "Man shapes himself through decisions that shape his environment."

Three Easy Steps

1. Decrease sources of toxicity. Remove the most glaring environmental pollutants in your home

2. Improve the body's own elimination process. Drink plenty of water and change to a diet that includes more fruit, vegetables and fiber.

3. Remove toxins already stored inside you. Do a cleansing fast once a month and consider investing in a far-infrared sauna.

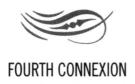

FOURTH CONNEXION

SUPPLEMENTATION

---

*To all my little Hulkamaniacs, say your prayers, take
your vitamins, and you will never go wrong.*

HULK HOGAN, CHAMPION PROFESSIONAL WRESTLER

The use of herbs and foods as medicines goes back as far as the
dawn of civilization. The Sumerians, who lived 6,000 years ago in
what is now Iraq, left clay tablets detailing the medicinal uses of
opium poppies, thyme, licorice and mustard plants. Chinese herbal
medicine has written records going back more than 3,000 years.
And long before vitamins were identified, the ancient Egyptians
already knew that eating liver would help cure night blindness,
which we now know is caused by Vitamin A deficiency.

In 1905, William Fletcher, an English doctor, made the important
discovery that beriberi, a disease common in Asia, could be
prevented by eating unpolished instead of polished rice. Seven
years later, in 1912, Casimir Funk, a biochemist working at the
Lister Institute in London, isolated the active substances in
unpolished rice husks that helped prevent beriberi. He called them
"vitamines" — from the Latin "vita," meaning life, and "amines,"
compounds derived from ammonia. When it was found that not all

vitamins were "amines," the "e" at the end was dropped and the name has been vitamins ever since.

Over the next several decades scientists isolated the actual vitamins and demonstrated their biochemical functions and their roles in preventing disease. The deprivation theory, that a lack of vitamins could make you sick, became widely accepted. As Nobel laureate Alfred Szent-Györgyi, who discovered Vitamin C, said, "A vitamin is a substance that makes you ill if you don't eat it."

In 1933, Vitamin C, also known as ascorbic acid, was first synthesized in a laboratory. (Ascorbic acid means "anti-scurvy," referring to its ability to cure scurvy, a deadly disease that had for centuries afflicted sailors on long ocean voyages.) Soon vitamins were commercially produced, and by the end of the decade, pharmaceutical companies were reaping large profits from vitamin sales.

Today, our understanding of vitamins and other substances, such as minerals, hormones and enzymes, continues to grow. As we deepen our knowledge of their important functions in the human body, we continue to expand the possibilities for greater health and well-being.

Vitamin Basics

Vitamins are small molecules which are necessary for life. With the exception of Vitamin D and Niacin, the body cannot synthesize vitamins on its own and must therefore get them from foods or food supplements. Of the 13 vitamins the body needs, four are fat soluble (A, D, E and K). The others are water soluble (all the B Vitamins, C, Panthothenic acid, and biotin).

A deficiency in just one vitamin can cause serious health problems. For example, a lack of Vitamin D causes rickets, a bone softening disease; not enough E leads to anemia; insufficient K can bring about internal bleeding; and a lack of B3 or Niacin causes pellagra, with symptoms that include skin sores, diarrhea, mental confusion and delusions.

But vitamins do much more than prevent disease. The B Vitamins — folic acid, B12 and B6, for example — are important for controlling levels of homocysteine (a sulfur-containing amino acid) in the blood. Their impact on health is significant, because elevated levels of homocysteine are associated with heart disease, atherosclerosis, stroke, Alzheimer's and osteoporosis.[1]

Just how powerful the effect of vitamins can be is demonstrated by the story of Eve Prang Plews. As a young woman in her twenties, she had vascular disease which caused frequent bruising. One day, she happened to come across a book by Linus Pauling that suggested that bruising is often the result of a Vitamin C deficiency. Four months after she started taking Vitamin C supplements, Plews slipped on the cement steps of her home. Expecting to wake up the next morning black and blue from ankle to thigh, she was surprised to find no bruises whatsoever. It was the first time in her life that Plews made the connection between vitamins and healing. She embarked on a career as a nutritional counselor, and has since helped numerous people improve their health through changes in diet and supplementation.

Minerals

Since the discoveries of vitamins and their functions, we have also learned about the importance of minerals and how they work in conjunction with vitamins. Minerals are elements essential to creating specific molecules which the body needs but cannot produce on its own. All minerals must come from outside sources, either from food or supplements.

Minerals become the hard substances of our bodies — bones, teeth and connective tissue. They are involved in most of the body's processes, including nerve transmission, muscle contraction and blood formation. In particular, they help manage the body's PH, keeping it from getting too alkaline or acidic. They also aid in the formation of antibodies and hormones that maintain the body's immune system.

Minerals essential to the body fall into two categories:

- Macrominerals that the body needs in large amounts: calcium, chloride, magnesium, potassium, sulfur and sodium.

- Microminerals or trace minerals that the body needs in small amounts: copper, iodine, iron, manganese, molybdenum, selenium and zinc.

As with vitamins, the lack of a particular mineral can cause serious health problems. Most people now know that insufficient calcium in bones will lead to osteoporosis. Other symptoms of calcium deficiency include diminished nerve functions, muscle cramping, insomnia, anxiety and depression.

Magnesium acts as a muscle relaxant in the body. It is an important nutrient for the heart, plays a role in hormone regulation, and enables the maintenance and repair of cells. A deficiency of this element leads to fatigue, gastrointestinal disorders, high blood pressure, irregular heartbeat, memory problems, mood swings and impaired motor skills.[2]

We continue to make new discoveries regarding the complex interactions of vitamins and minerals and their effect on the body.

The Current State of Dietary Supplements

For a long time, "dietary supplements" meant vitamins and minerals. But in 1994, Congress passed the Dietary Supplement Health and Education Act (DSHEA), expanding the definition to include herbs, other botanicals (except tobacco) and any substance used to augment the diet.

DSHEA led to many other supplements coming onto the market, including amino acids, fiber (like psyllium and guar gum), and compounds not normally considered foods or nutrients, such as hormones and enzymes. Soon after DSHEA's passage, annual sales of dietary supplements jumped from $4 billion to $12 billion, because manufacturers were no longer required to seek approval from the Food and Drug Administration (FDA) to bring a new product on the market. What once was an industry requiring FDA approval has become a virtually unregulated business. You yourself could chop up a bunch of herbs, put them in a bottle and make claims of their effectiveness.

Step inside any health food store, supermarket or drug store, and you will find shelves crammed full of nutraceuticals promising all kinds of health benefits. Surveys show that more than half of American adults take supplements to augment their diet. Yet few know how accurate their claims are.

As a result, many medical doctors, skeptical of unsubstantiated claims, do not recommend supplementation. As far as getting the necessary vitamins and minerals, they offer the age-old prescription that "Eating a healthy diet will provide all the nutrition you need." While we are very much in favor of eating right, we do not believe that it is possible to obtain all of the nutrition the body needs for proper functioning from food alone.

The Need for Supplementation

There are several reasons why just eating a balanced diet is not enough. According to statistics compiled by the U.S. Department of Agriculture, between 1900 and 1980:

- fresh fruit and vegetable consumption decreased from 40 percent to five percent

- whole grain consumption decreased 50 percent

- fresh apple consumption decreased 70 percent

- beef consumption increased 75 percent

- cheese consumption increased 400 percent

- fat and oil consumption increased 150 percent

- margarine consumption increased 800 percent

Not a pretty picture.

Even if you decide to improve your eating habits, there is no guarantee that the foods you eat contain any nutritional value. We have all experienced the bland taste of tomatoes that have been engineered to harden the skin so that machines can pick them. Plants cannot obtain minerals from depleted soils. You would have to eat 50 cans of spinach today to equal the amount of nutrients in one can in 1950![3]

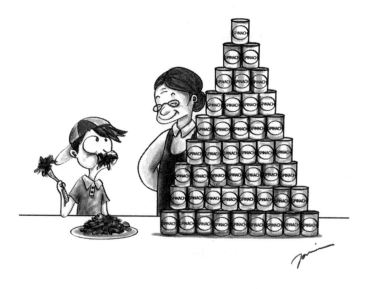

"Do I have to eat all of those?"

Many fruits and vegetables are treated with pesticides, herbicides, and hormones. Dairy products and meats contain growth hormones and antibiotics.

Processed Food

Consumption of processed foods has had a dramatic effect on the health of Americans. Remember the beriberi story. It is polished (processed) rice that leads to the vitamin deficiency that causes the disease. There are 40 nutrients that cannot be made in the body. In addition to vitamins and minerals, they include essential fatty acids and amino acids. Processing removes or kills most of the natural fiber and nutrients contained in food.

At the same time, chemical preservatives are added to increase the shelf life of food by controlling the growth of molds and bacteria. Other common methods of preservation include pasteurization (heating), sterilization, irradiation, freezing and canning. All of them are designed to kill microbes. In the process, they also eliminate most of what is valuable and nutritious.

The Case of Enzymes

Consider the impact on enzymes, for example. Enzymes are proteins that regulate chemical reactions in the body. Without enzymes there is no life. But heating any food above 122 degrees Fahrenheit destroys any live enzyme activity. Thus, processed foods contain virtually no enzymes.

Enzymes come either from outside food sources — raw vegetables and fruits — or are manufactured by the body. Without enzymes the body is unable to digest food. Witness the huge market in pills, powders and liquids sold to combat indigestion. When our digestive system is compromised, we do not process thoroughly what we eat. On average, people digest less than 70 percent of the food they take in.

When it lacks digestive enzymes, the body steals amino acids from other organs, which affects their functions. Hair and skin may become dry, resulting in premature aging. More seriously, the liver is unable to handle the excretion of waste products, resulting in exhaustion, weakening of the immune system, and a greater susceptibility to degenerative diseases. According to an article in "Today's Health," a magazine published by the American Medical Association, researchers now believe that many diseases can be traced to enzyme deprivation.

Pottinger's Cats

During the 1940s, a medical doctor named Francis Pottinger conducted a study to determine the effect of processed food on the body. He studied 900 cats over several generations, dividing them into five groups. Each group was fed one of the following: raw milk, pasteurized milk, evaporated milk and condensed milk. All groups received a minimal diet required to sustain life.

The two groups of cats raised on raw food remained healthy through four generations. The three groups of cats supplied with processed milk, however, developed degenerative health conditions, including arthritis, allergies and diabetes, toward the end of their lives. The second generation cats showed the same diseases during the middle of their lives. The third generation cats had them at the beginning of their lives, and many died before they were six months old. There was no fourth generation, because so many of the third generation parents were sterile or aborted their offspring before birth.

For purposes of health and wellness, it is significant that the trend in human health is following Dr. Pottinger's results rather closely. Since the introduction of processed food, degenerative and immune system-related diseases are on the rise. Several generations later, children now are either born with degenerative diseases or develop them much earlier in life. Conception levels have decreased in all Western countries, and miscarriages are increasing.[4]

While the relationship between processed food and poor health is a complex matter, more and more studies are pointing to the benefits of whole, natural, organic foods over their processed and synthetically manufactured counterparts.

Enriched Food

Because processing and preserving destroys most nutrients, the food industry has developed "enriched" foods, adding synthetic vitamins and minerals to make up for the depletion. During the refining of flour for commercial breads and cereals, for example, most of the B and E vitamins, biotin and panthothenic acid are discarded. To make up for this loss, the synthetic versions of these vitamins are added. The resulting products are labeled as "enriched" or "fortified," and marketed as offering health and wellness benefits.

There is considerable controversy, however, regarding the effectiveness of synthetic vs. natural vitamins, derived from whole foods. One side argues that vitamin molecules are identical whether they are produced in a chemical laboratory or from a natural plant. The other side contends that not all vitamins are alike. Vitamins produced from whole foods are a combination of components — enzymes, co-enzymes and co-factors — that make absorption easier and work together to produce the intended biochemical effects. Studies have shown, for example, that consumption of natural, rather than synthetic, Vitamin E produced higher and longer lasting levels in the blood.[5]

While more research is needed, we believe that the way vitamins operate in the human body is a complex process that is best served by natural products. Natural whole-food supplements offer many wellness benefits not available from synthetics.

As We Grow Older

As we age, the lining in our intestines absorbs fewer nutrients from the food we eat. Our organs don't function as well, and our skin loses some of its capacity to create Vitamin D. Studies have shown that the skin of elderly people is only 40 percent as efficient as a child's skin.[6]

Because older people tend to eat less than younger people, they also take in fewer vitamins and minerals at the very time when they actually need more. Studies have demonstrated, for example, that Vitamin E enhances immune system function, which is often compromised among the elderly.[7]

Supplementation

For all of the above reasons, we believe that supplementation is essential for health and wellness.

Yet there is much confusion, given the wealth of information and numerous supplements available in the market. How can you tell which of the many brands to buy? What is natural rather than synthetic? What are the necessary minimum daily requirements? To simplify, we have identified five areas of supplementation and some basic advice on each.

General Health

Bone health

Heart health

Cleansing health

Anti-Aging Health

GENERAL HEALTH

In addition to eating right, we recommend **taking a daily multiple vitamin and mineral supplement** made from whole foods. For people under 30, a complete, natural multivitamin will supply all the essential additional nutrients required. For those older than 30, more supplementation is advisable.

When selecting a multivitamin, be sure to choose a supplement that provides at least 100 percent of the daily recommended minimums (RDAs — recommended dietary allowances) in most or all categories.

Invest some time and research into finding a good supplement. Pay special attention to how easily it can be absorbed. Thomas Brobeil, the city manager of Gulfport, Florida, was inspecting the city's waste management facility when he noticed a sea of small colored pellets clogging a screen. One of the workers told him, smiling, that they were vitamins pills whose coating was so hard that they had gone through people undigested.

BONE HEALTH

As the most abundant mineral in the body, the role of **calcium** in building and maintaining strong, healthy bones is undisputed — almost 99 percent of it occurs in bone tissues. The rest maintains normal heart beat, regulates blood pressure, and aids in the functioning of the nervous system. A constant supply of calcium is necessary throughout life, but it is especially important for women during pregnancy and breast feeding. As we grow older, it is essential to supplement with calcium to keep bones strong and to prevent osteoporosis.

The standard American diet is estimated to supply only one-third of our daily calcium needs. The recommended daily intake for adults is 1,000-1,200 mgs, but women need as much as 1,500 mgs a day. Many daily multivitamin tablets supply much less than that, so additional calcium supplements may be necessary.[8]

Because of its recent popularity, there are many calcium products on the market, some with outrageous claims — one infomercial for coral calcium suggested that it can cure 200 diseases. Don't buy the excessive hype, but don't let it turn you away from this essential, life-giving mineral either.

Calcium absorption depends on a number of factors, including the acidity of the lower intestine, Vitamin D and estrogen levels in the body, and the type of calcium supplement. Calcium carbonate, for example, is widely available and inexpensive, but poorly absorbed. We recommend calcium citrate or calcium gluconate (or a combination of both), preferably in the form of effervescent powder, which is highly bio-available in the digestive tract. Because magnesium aids calcium absorption, we recommend supplements that combine the two.

HEART HEALTH

We have already mentioned the power of **omega-3, omega-6** and **essential fatty acids (EFAs)**, which support the reproductive, immune and nervous systems. For Americans struggling with heart disease and obesity, the role of EFAs in cardiovascular health is critical. These "good fats" raise good cholesterol (HDL) levels and help break down bad cholesterol (LDL), undoing some of the damage done by saturated and killer fats.

Most Americans can get enough omega-6 (linoleic acid) from their diet, especially if they use olive oil on a regular basis. But they are likely to be deficient in omega-3 (linolenic acid). Flaxseed is a good source of omega-3. Fish such as salmon, trout and albacore tuna are others. But high heat destroys linolenic acid, so cooked fish does not provide omega-3 in sufficient amounts.[9] We recommend daily supplements of omega-3 from fish oil in capsule form that is guaranteed free of mercury.

CLEANSING HEALTH

Antioxidants help eliminate free radicals. In the process, they cleanse the body of inflammation, increase immune functions, and help decrease the risk of infection and cancer.

Some of the better known antioxidants are Vitamins C and E, and the minerals magnesium, copper and zinc. Be aware of the relationship between the last two. Zinc taken alone leaches copper from the body, so taking either a combination zinc-copper supplement or additional copper is advisable.

Other food compounds are the carotenoids — precursors of Vitamin A — such as beta-carotene and lycopene. Apricots, broccoli, pumpkin, cantaloupes, spinach and sweet potatoes are good sources of beta-carotene. Lycopene, the pigment that gives tomatoes and watermelon their red color, also seems to have powerful antioxidant qualities.[10] Studies suggest that consuming foods rich in lycopene is associated with a lower risk of prostate cancer.[11] In fact, all colorful fruits or vegetables have high antioxidant qualities.

You can get many antioxidant benefits by eating right and taking a good daily vitamin and mineral supplement. We also recommend taking CoQ10, a coenzyme that occurs naturally in the body and is critical in the production of energy for each cell. It is one of the most powerful antioxidant supplements.

ANTI-AGING HEALTH

One of the most exciting developments in supplementation has been the discovery that **human growth hormone** can reverse the aging process. After men and women reach their thirties, growth hormone levels in their bodies start to fall, diminishing with every decade. Replacing it can slow down, halt, and even reverse many of the symptoms we associate with growing old. Originally used to combat dwarfism, growth hormones became a fad in the 1980s and 90s when a number of media stars went to Mexico to receive injections of animal hormones on a regular basis. The treatment was expensive — over $10,000 a month — and had dangerous side effects. In recent years a natural, purified source of HGH has become available, which is more affordable and safer, costing as little as $300 a month.

There is, however, an even less expensive alternative: **Human Growth Hormone(HGH) Secretagogue** (a secretagogue is an agent that causes or stimulates secretion). HGH Secretagogue is composed of amino acids that are precursors of HGH. Instead of injecting a foreign substance, HGH Secretagogue works by stimulating the pituitary gland to secrete the body's own human growth hormone.

HGH Secretagogue builds muscle mass throughout the body. Other benefits include weight loss, increased energy levels, improved memory and vision, increase in bone mass, and a strengthened immune system. It is also one of the best providers of natural face lifts. Firming up tissue, building muscle, and restoring skin elasticity counters all the wrinkle developments that come with aging.[12]

The cancer potential in taking HGH Secretagogue is a controversial subject. Some people feel that it is possible, since the genesis of cancer cells is excessive growth. There is an opposite view that HGH Secretagogue actually decreases the risk of cancer, since people rarely get cancer in their 20s and 30s when human growth hormone levels are at their highest. Although there has been never been a case which even suggests that HGH Secretagogue has caused or contributed to cancer, we recommend that if you have a family history of cancer, have or have had cancer, you should discuss this with your personal physician before taking such products.

A Sensible Approach

While there are other supplements available for specific health issues, space does not permit us to discuss all of them. There are literally thousands of dietary supplements on the market, enough to fill several books. Let us instead offer some basic guidelines.

- Approach too-good-to-be-true claims with healthy skepticism. Remember that "natural" does not automatically mean "safe" or "good for you." Opium and heroin are both natural products.

- Find out what side effects supplements may have. Some herbals interfere with pharmaceutical or over-the-counter drugs and can cause serious complications. Be sure to tell your doctor what you are taking, especially if you are hospitalized.

- Do not exceed the recommended daily dosage unless suggested by a physician. High doses of some supplements can be harmful. Too much Vitamin A causes toxic responses. The ephedra scandal a few years ago resulted from the unregulated use of the ancient Chinese herb. When several people, including Baltimore Orioles pitcher Steve Bechler, died after taking supplements containing ephedra, the FDA banned the substance.

- Supplementation doesn't make up for poor nutritional choices. Be sure to include plenty of colorful fruits and vegetables in your diet.

- Supplementation is not a miracle cure. If you are chronically ill, taking prescription drugs, or are pregnant or breastfeeding, consult with a physician or holistic medical doctor before taking any supplements.

Do not let these caveats discourage you from using supplementation to enhance your health and well-being. While it may take some time to settle on the right supplements for you, the benefits over time are well worth it.

Three Easy Steps

1. Take a daily multivitamin/mineral supplement.

2. Take a daily calcium supplement.

3. Take daily omega-3 from fish in capsule form.

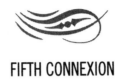

FIFTH CONNEXION

EXERCISE

A bear, however hard he tries, grows tubby without exercise.

A.A. MILNE, POOH'S LITTLE INSTRUCTION BOOK

America seems to be riding the wave of a fitness craze. Health clubs are popping up across the country like convenience stores, providing opportunities for workouts at all times of the day. In 2003 and 2004, Curves for Women, offering 30-minute exercise sessions on a variety of machines, was the second fastest growing franchise in the United States and Canada.[1] In many suburbs, you can see people walking or jogging in the mornings and after work. Walking in air-conditioned malls has become a popular pastime among retirees in Southern states when the temperature outside gets too hot.

But are these signs of a new dawn of American fitness? Hardly. If that were the case, obesity would not be on the rise at epidemic rates for all age groups. In the computer age, most people live sedentary lives. They get into their cars to drive 300 feet to the supermarket. Their favorite activity is exercising their thumbs on the remote control for televisions and video games. As for all those supposed health club fanatics, it turns out that 90 percent of the people who sign up for memberships never make it much beyond their first workout. They end up following the example of Mark

Twain, the American humorist who said, "I have never taken any exercise, except sleeping and resting."

This sad state of affairs is true even though the benefits of exercising have been known for centuries. Over 2,000 years ago, Pliny the Younger, a lawyer and scientist in ancient Rome, noted, "It is remarkable how one's wits are sharpened by physical exercise." These days, there is practically unanimous agreement among scientists and doctors about the value of exercising.

Exercise provides all kinds of health benefits. It helps lower blood pressure, elevates "good" cholesterol (HDL), which the body needs, and reduces the "bad" (LDL) cholesterol that clogs arteries and causes heart disease.[2] Regular exercise can prevent or delay diseases like cancer, stroke and diabetes.[3] It is no accident that health organizations like the American Heart Association and the American Arthritis Foundation recommend exercising three to five times a week.

Want to manage your weight? There is no better way to stay fit and trim than leading an active life and drinking lots of water. According to the Fitness Fundamentals developed by the President's Council on Physical Fitness, "The combination of exercise and diet offers the most flexible and effective approach to weight control."

People who exercise feel better, look younger and sleep more soundly. Exercise can act as an antidote to depression. When you get your heart pumping, your brain releases chemicals called endorphins, which lift your mood and chase the doldrums away.

So what's the problem? Considering the almost universal accolades for the benefits of exercise, why do so few Americans do it? If it is the fountain of youth, why don't more people get on the program? Why do they prefer to follow in the footsteps of the American educator Robert M. Hutchins, who said, "Whenever I feel like exercise, I lie down until the feeling passes"? Have we simply become a lazy nation, in which people treat their bodies like rental cars — using them to get around, but caring little for their upkeep?

Perhaps one of the reasons that people avoid exercise is that they do not believe they will enjoy it. It sounds too much like hard work and effort for people who want to have fun and pursue pleasure. In the words of Oprah Winfrey, "There is no easy way out. If there was, I would have bought it. And believe me, it would be one of my favorite things."

Add to that a slew of myths about exercise, and it is no surprise that many people are afraid of doing something that would be good for them.

Cutting Through Excuses

Let's look at some of those myths.

NO PAIN, NO GAIN

This is simply not true. There is no need to work so hard that you have to grunt or scream like a tennis star attacking the ball. You don't have to do reps until your arms feel like they are going to fall off. In fact, if you feel more than minor discomfort, you are probably doing something wrong and should stop immediately! While it is always recommended to check with a physician before getting started, there is virtually no situation in which in some form of exercise will not improve a person's life.

At the urging of his wife, Marty became a patient of Dr. Watts. He had retired early because he had no energy and was depressed all the time. He had a mean, grouchy disposition and was so unfriendly that another doctor had put him on Prozac just so that he could get along with others.

When Dr. Watts suggested a change in diet and an exercise regimen, Marty claimed that, except for golf, he had never exercised before and did not believe in it. He began with a very basic exercise routine — about 15-20 minutes in the morning — doing calisthenics and working with light weights. Soon he began to lose weight and feel better. When his depression cleared, he turned out to be a charming man, so much so that he became a favorite of Dr. Watts' staff. After a year of basic good health, he took up golf again (knocking six strokes off his handicap), started a small business and went off Prozac because, as he said, he didn't need it any more.

I HAVE NO TIME

This is the favorite excuse of busy people. At a time when we are stressed and overworked, many feel that they simply cannot free up a few hours a week to work out. Yet, studies show that people who do take the time to exercise are more alert and focused and show greater productivity at work than those who try to boost their energy artificially with caffeine or other stimulants. To those who say that they can't afford to take the time to excercise, we say, "You really can't afford not to."

Exercise Is a Must

There is really no way around it: if you wish to enjoy a better quality of life, you have to exercise. Like an engine which gets sluggish and inefficient when it sits still too long, your body gets rusty and stagnates from inactivity. As Jimmy Connors, the tennis star, once said, "Use it, or lose it."

For an aging population, exercise is essential. As we get older, we tend to lose lean muscle tissue, which affects our strength, posture, balance and mobility. Yet much of this muscle loss can be slowed down and even reversed. The right kinds of exercise can make us feel younger than our biological age.[4]

Consider Hall of Fame baseball pitcher Nolan Ryan. Among his many achievements are most strikeouts (5,714) and fastest recorded pitch (100.9 miles an hour). He won 324 games, of which an astonishing seven were no-hitters. Remarkably, Ryan pitched his last two no-hitters at age 42 and 43. When asked how he managed to stay on top of the game for so long, he attributed his longevity to good throwing mechanics and regular exercise. He had a relentless work ethic, doing weight training every day.

Even for those of us who are not elite athletes, exercising is really just a mindset. It requires making a decision to do the things that will benefit your body and then taking action. The good news is that regular exercise is not nearly as difficult as many make it out to be. It doesn't have to be a chore. It can be as fun and enjoyable as it is rewarding.

Most people think of exercising only as jogging or working out at the gym — both repetitious activities that are boring. But there are many other forms, such as gardening, bike riding, dancing and — believe it or not — house work.

Let's get creative in our daily lives. Consider taking stairs instead of the elevator at work, getting up from your desk from time to time to stretch and walk around, carrying your own groceries, and parking at the far end of the mall parking lot instead of right in front of the entrance. You could learn a new sport or game, rake leaves or take tango lessons.

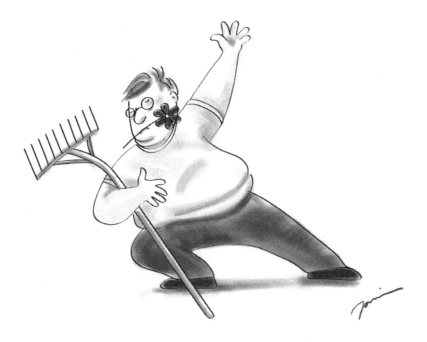

Exercise can be fun.

So, why not get going? The only thing you have to lose — is some weight.

Getting Started

Many people who want to get started exercising don't know what steps to take. There is such a wealth of information available about exercise on the Internet, in videos and in books, that the sheer volume can be daunting. For this reason, we have put together a primer on what you need to know if you want to embark on an exercise program that will improve your health and quality of life.

There are three types of exercise:

- aerobic or cardiovascular conditioning

- weight or resistance training

- stretching or flexibility training

Let's examine each of them in more detail.

Aerobic Exercise

Aerobic means "with air," so aerobic exercise is an activity that requires oxygen and increases the intake of air. It is also called cardiovascular exercise, from Latin for "heart" and "vessel," because it increases blood circulation. As we exercise, we need more air, forcing the heart to pump faster and send more blood flowing through the body. Since the heart is fundamentally a muscle, regular aerobic workouts will improve its ability to do its job.

Brisk walking, jogging, running, bicycling, swimming, cross-country skiing, rowing, jumping rope and roller-blading are all true aerobic exercises that can raise your heart rate over a continuous period of time.

All of these activities need to be done at a moderate pace. Extremely vigorous exercise can create an oxygen debt, resulting in a buildup of lactic acid in the muscles, defeating the purpose of the exercise. A good rule of thumb to follow is: You should be mildly out of breath at all times, but not wheezing. If you can comfortably sing or talk while doing the activity — great. Otherwise, you need to slow down.

Another simple way to monitor your level of exercise is to check your pulse. The appropriate aerobic rate is roughly 180 minus your age. So if you are 55 years old, your ideal pulse rate would be 180 minus 55, or 125. You can check your pulse by placing the tips of your fingers lightly on one of the blood vessels in your neck or the inside of your wrist below the thumb. Be sure to check your heart rate within five seconds of stopping the exercise, because it will quickly drop to its normal baseline.

When you start out with your program, check your pulse from time to time to make sure you are exercising without exceeding your target heart rate. It is okay to be well below that. As you get in better shape, you will be able to stay close to your age-appropriate aerobic threshold.

If you are taking any medicines or have an illness that changes your natural heart rate (for example beta blockers, which regulate blood pressure), consult with your doctor before starting on any kind of exercise regimen.

Decide what form of exercise works best for you. You may agree with Thomas Jefferson, the third U.S. president, that "... of all the exercises walking is the best." Walking actually provides 90 percent of the health benefits of running. If you have knee problems, the impact on the road, sidewalk or treadmill when jogging or running might not be good for you. Even brisk walking can cause joint pain. You might find bicycling or swimming more to your liking (but not in chlorinated pools). Some gyms have elliptical machines that reduce the stress on ankles and knees.

Study after study has demonstrated that aerobic exercise is one of the most effective ways of lowering blood pressure, reducing the risk of heart attacks, toning muscles, controlling stress and trimming fat.[5]

Losing weight requires burning 3,500 more calories than you take in just to get rid of one pound.

Below is a chart of the approximate number of calories burned per hour in various aerobic exercises by a person weighing 100, 150 and 200 pounds.

Activity	100 lbs	150 lbs	200 lbs
Bicycling, 6 mph	160	240	312
Bicycling, 12 mph	270	410	534
Jogging, 7 mph	610	920	1,230
Jumping Rope	500	750	1,000
Running, 5.5mph	440	660	962
Running, 10 mph	850	1,280	1,664
Swimming, 25 yds/min	185	275	358
Swimming, 50 yds/min	325	500	650
Walking, 2 mph	160	240	312
Walking, 3 mph	210	320	416
Walking, 4.5 mph	295	440	572

Source: American Heart Association

According to the above chart, if you weigh 150 pounds, you would have to walk about 30 miles to burn 3,500 calories. You can do that in 10 hours in one day, or spread it out one mile a day for 30 days. The average person takes about 3,000 steps each day just in the normal course of daily activity. If you can raise that to 10,000 steps a day, you will be well on your way to taking off those extra pounds.

Roger Ebert, the "thumbs up" movie critic, accomplishes that by monitoring his steps during the day. He wears a small pedometer hooked to his belt — you can buy one for around $12 to $15 — and when he finds that it is getting late in the afternoon or evening, and he has not reached the 10,000 mark, he kicks in a bit extra.

Conscious, aerobic exercise provides a good return for the time invested. It can improve sleep, decreasing the time needed for restorative slumber, and increase energy throughout the day. So if you think you feel too tired to walk, jog or swim, think again. Break the cycle of inactivity and start experiencing a renewed flow of energy.

Resistance Training

Resistance or weight training involves pushing or pulling against something that makes muscles exert themselves. Working out with free weights or weight machines are the most popular and well-known examples. But our own bodies can provide ample resistance in exercises such as push-ups, pull-ups, squats, calisthenics and rope climbing, or in games such as tug-of-war.

An inexpensive alternative to joining a health club or investing in free weight equipment to use at home are therabands (short for therapeutic bands) — heavy-duty, elastic rubber strips that can be attached to doorways or furniture and used to exercise all the major muscle groups. Therabands come in a variety of colors, indicating the different amount of resistance they offer, and cover a wide variety of effective strengthening exercises.

Resistance training is the most effective form of exercise for burning fat. Unlike aerobic exercise, it burns calories during the activity and afterward. As muscle fibers are being rebuilt after exercise, our metabolic rates stay elevated (after aerobic workouts they quickly return quickly to normal). As a result of this "after-burn," many calories we consume later in the day will be used up instead of being stored as fat.

The human body consumes between 30 to 50 calories per pound of muscle per day. Thus, every pound of muscle you add results in an increase in the amount of calories your body needs to function. The more muscle tissue you have, the more calories your body will consume, even on the days you do not exercise. Of course, the increase in lean muscle and elimination of unsightly bulges will make you look and feel better as well.

It used to be thought that the body stopped growing at a certain age. But studies show that weight training can lead to an increase in human growth hormone (HGH) levels even in 60 and 70 year olds. When subjects lifted weights at 70 percent of their maximum capacity, HGH levels tripled. At 85 percent of maximum capacity, they quadrupled![6]

Resistance training also increases bone density, good news for those suffering from osteoporosis, which makes bones more fragile. Osteoporosis can lead to increased fractures and excessive curvature of the spine. Weight training helps prevent or stop the development of this debilitating disease, common in menopausal women. Working out with weights can also cause a significant increase in bone mineral content, which can be maintained with continued training as people get older.[7]

Above all, weight training makes you stronger, regardless of gender or age. With a good regimen, most people get stronger in a matter of weeks. An increase in muscle strength tends to reduce injuries, especially in older people. If your leg and hip muscles are strong, they provide a solid foundation and support, making it less likely that you will fall. And even if you do, you will be more likely to be able to get up on your own.

Flexibility Training

Most of us, when we wake up in the morning, stretch in bed. It feels good and works the kinks out of our bodies after a night's sleep. Yet we often treat stretching and flexibility training as an afterthought — something to do during warm-up and cooling down phases of the "real" workout. Stretching itself is an important exercise. Many physical trainers suggest that being flexible should be the main goal of working out.

Flexibility can be defined as "the range of possible motion around a joint." Gentle activities such as yoga, tai chi or pilates, and more rigorous pursuits like martial arts, ballet, tumbling and gymnastics, all increase flexibility. Television exercise programs usually include stretching routines.

Flexibility exercise should be done slowly, breathing in while getting to the point of resistance and breathing out while relaxing into the stretch. Never bounce to increase flexibility, because you could tear ligaments. Instead, ease into it gradually and let gravity do the work.

The reason stretching is so important is that our normal daily activities do not even come close to moving our joints through their full range of motion. Many people, by the time they are teenagers, are already severely limited, unable to touch their toes or lean backward with natural agility. Stiff and tight muscles affect posture. They are the most common cause of lower back pain. Studies show that stretching programs more than any other type of therapy get the best results in relieving chronic back pain.[8]

Stretching is also one of the best ways to relief stress. Our muscles become chronically tense, wasting energy and requiring extra exertion, making us more tired and irritable. As stretching relaxes these muscles, it makes them less susceptible to fatigue and pain.

Imagine the number of pain pills we would not need to take for headaches, backaches, upset stomachs and sleeplessness if we heeded the advice of the American Arthritis Foundation and stretched every day!

Do All Three

Doing any of these three forms of exercise on a regular basis will lead to significant improvement in the way you look, feel and engage the world. But the best results will happen if you combine all three categories in a well-balanced exercise program.

Regular exercise will increase the quality of your life dramatically, improving health, boosting energy and providing a greater sense of well-being. Improved stamina will increase productivity. Weight loss and improved appearance will enhance your self-image, encouraging you to seek out new acquaintances with confidence and to engage in a wider range of activities with family and friends.

A Simple Routine

Here is a simple, easy to follow exercise routine that covers all the bases. It takes **only one hour, three times a week.**

- 10 minutes warm-up by stretching,

- 20 minutes weight training,

- 20 minutes aerobic exercise,

- 10 minutes cool down by stretching.

For a shorter daily program, 40 minutes five times a week, alternate weight training and aerobic exercise each day:

- 10 minutes warm-up by stretching

- 20 minutes weight training **or** aerobic exercise

- 10 minutes cool down by stretching

Try to schedule exercise at the same time — before work, during lunch or at night. Repetition and consistency establish habits. Convenience and a reasonable schedule will make it easier to stick to the routine.

Some Dos and Don'ts

- Wear comfortable clothes and shoes.

- Drink lots of filtered water before, during and after each exercise period.

- For outdoor exercise, avoid the hot and humid times of the day.

- Don't hold your breath while straining to lift a weight. It may seem counter-intuitive, but it is best to breathe out while your muscles are working and breathe in when they relax.

- Stop at the first sign of muscle cramping, dizziness, chest pain, shortness of breath or palpitations (heart racing). Exercise should not hurt or exhaust you. A little soreness, some mild discomfort, a bit of weariness are all normal. But you should not feel pain.

- Don't compare yourself to others. Exercising is not a contest but a way of life that must make sense to you. A doctor at the Mayo Clinic in Rochester, Minnesota, had an obese patient so heavy she could not get out of a wheelchair. He worked with her to stand up three times a day. From there, she graduated to walking 15 seconds at a time. Getting to walk for two minutes was a major victory.

She might have never made progress if she had compared herself to a marathon runner.

- If you decide to join a gym or health club, find one close to your home or place of work. If you have to travel across town to get there, your commitment will likely decrease soon after joining.

- Integrate exercise into your everyday life. Make it part of your daily routine. Studies show that people who do their exercising at the same time each day stay with the program longer than people who fit it in whenever possible.

- Pursue such non-glamorous activities as taking stairs, raking leaves, carrying your own grocery bags, and walking. Be nice to your car and park in the back of the lot, away from other vehicles. Walking the extra distance to your destination will make a difference.

- Take your time. Be patient. Don't expect immediate results. Too many people have an all-or-nothing mentality. After years of doing nothing, they get inspired, play basketball or jog several miles, develop shin splints, pulled muscles or sprained ankles, and then go right back to doing nothing, worse off than they were before. Don't be a weekend warrior who has to nurse his aches and pains throughout the week.

- Set reasonable goals, and be sure to reward yourself when you attain them.

Having Fun

Make exercise a fun, positive experience. If you are a walker, take along a headset and listen to music or books on tape. Susan, a home business owner, works out regularly, but hates weight machines. "How many times can you count to 16 without wanting to scream," she says. But she loves aerobic classes or any other class that includes music.

Some people like to work out with people, others hate crowds. Some like working out in the comfort of a home gym first thing in the morning with therabands and hand weights, while others prefer lunch time or evening. Whatever works best for you and makes exercising an enjoyable experience is golden. If it is pleasurable, you will give it enough time to start working. Once it works, the results will keep you motivated to keep going.

For most people, it takes only a few hours a week to bring about improved health and well-being. It may change your life!

So here is the way to get started:

- Choose an activity appropriate to your lifestyle. If you suffer from a hernia, weight lifting is not a good option. Therabands are a gentler approach. They may also be more appealing to women who don't like to work out with heavy weights.

- if you like to work out with other people, join a health club. Find a partner for motivation and socializing. The buddy system can work wonders.

- If you can afford it, hire a certified personal trainer. Some of them will come to your house; others work only at health clubs. In either case, the combination of making an appointment and paying for it will add to your motivation.

- Be accountable to someone. Involve your family to cheer you on or keep you on track.

- Rent a few exercise videos from your local library or video store and find the ones you like best. Then buy them so you can work out in the comfort of your home.

- Go step by step, rather than all at once. Start slowly and build up over time to greater strength, flexibility and stamina.

- Visualize your goals and see yourself as having reached

them. You will only go as far as your self-image allows.

- Schedule rest days.

- Pay attention to your body. If you feel faint, have difficulty breathing, get chest pains or experience palpitations, stop immediately and see a physician. If you suffer from any chronic illnesses or take pharmaceutical drugs on a regular basis, be sure to check with your doctor before beginning any exercise program.

A Final Caution

Although exercise is essential for good health, it is not a cure-all. Do not make it the only area in your life where you practice wellness. Studies show, for example, that if you are fat, it does not matter if you are fit.[10] Just because someone who is overweight can play basketball or run around a baseball field — demonstrating aerobic fitness — does not necessarily diminish the risk of cardiovascular disease. Remember, all the jogging Bill Clinton did during his presidency did not prevent him from having to undergo heart bypass surgery later on.

Exercising is only one of many important wellness principles.

Three Easy Steps

1. Make a decision to start exercising.

2. Choose an activity that you enjoy and that fits your lifestyle.

3. Do it at least three times a week.

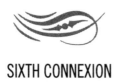

SIXTH CONNEXION

STRESS MANAGEMENT

Stress is an ignorant state. It believes that everything is an emergency.

NATALIE GOLDBERG, AMERICAN WRITER

Like death and taxes, stress is an inevitable part of life. From the daily grind and time pressures of modern life to traumatic events, such as the death of a loved one, a serious illness or the loss of a job, stress takes its toll on our health and well-being. Major man-made and natural disasters such as 9-11 and Hurricane Katrina result in post-traumatic stress disorder on a large scale, with a host of debilitating symptoms and conditions for those who suffer from it.

But not all stress is negative. Marriage, pregnancy, birthday parties, and visits by good friends or relatives all can be both positive and stressful. Stress also propels people to take action, become more productive and creative, and make new, exciting discoveries. Thrill seekers welcome the stress of roller-coaster rides, sky diving and competitive sports. Without some stress, life would be a dull affair, indeed, which led Hans Selye, an endocrinologist and the father of stress research, to insist that "Stress is the spice of life."

A Historical Perspective

Stress is the body's way of reacting to threatening situations in order to survive. In prehistoric times, when external threats were a matter of life and death, stress gave humans extra energy to escape or fight predators. This so-called "fight or flight" reaction releases stress hormones that "pump up" the body in anticipation of doing battle or running away.

In today's world, we no longer confront saber-tooth tigers and woolly mammoths. Our dangers are usually more psychological — traffic jams, work deadlines, demanding bosses and arguments with spouse or children.

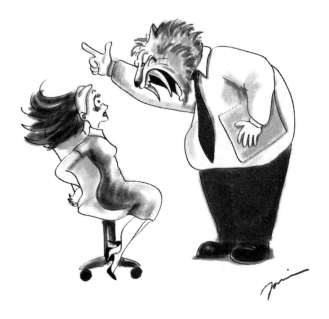

His bark is worse than his bite.

The problem is that our bodies respond to these perceived threats with the same fight or flight mechanism.[1] As a result, stress hormones are released even when we do not need them to protect us. In the process, they affect our health, and over time make us more vulnerable to serious illnesses.[2]

Fortunately, there are ways to manage stress. Once we become aware of the symptoms and some of the underlying causes, we can begin to cope with stress in a positive way that can lead to improved health and well-being, and even to a longer life.

Two Kinds of Stress

The body's hormonal reaction can be beneficial in dealing with **acute** stressful situations, but **chronic** stress can cause serious health consequences.

Most of us recognize the symptoms of acute stress in response to an immediate crisis, such as a fender bender or a heated argument. Heart rate and blood pressure rise; palms feel sweaty or cold. We might experience dizziness, shortness of breath and chest pains. Our muscles tense, causing headaches and back pain. Gastrointestinal symptoms can include heartburn, diarrhea and constipation. We may also feel mental distress, including the three stress emotions — anger, anxiety and depression.

Once the crisis has passed, the body recovers. Our heart rate, blood pressure and metabolism return to normal. Many people feel exhausted and even nod off for a while. A good night's sleep aids the recovery process. In fact, sleep is one of the best anti-aging and stress relief activities.

The Problem of Chronic Stress

Chronic stress occurs when we endure stressful situations without the opportunity to fully recover. Many people in demanding jobs, unhappy relationships or financial difficulties live in a never-ending cycle of tension and stress. In our modern life, we are exposed to many more stressful situations than our prehistoric ancestors ever had to face, including environmental triggers such as elevated noise levels and chemical pollution.

The result is a steady activation of the body's stress response system, the long-term effects of which are damaging to our health.

Chronic stress increases the risk of obesity, ulcers, heart disease and perhaps even cancer. The two most used pharmaceutical drugs in the U.S. are for digestive problems and headaches, which are directly linked to stress. According to Harvard Medical School Professor Herbert Benson, M.D., "Experts now believe that that 60 to 90 percent of all doctor visits involve stress-related complaints." [3]

Perhaps the most dangerous aspect of chronic stress is that many people are unaware of its impact on their lives. They have grown so accustomed to it that they do not recognize that their mood swings, irritability, forgetfulness, loss of concentration, feelings of anxiety, fatigue, depression, low self-esteem, and lack of interest in life all may have stress as their root cause.[4]

How Stress Affects the Body

When we feel physically or psychologically threatened, our body goes on red alert. The pituitary gland, located at the base of the brain, discharges extra hormones that signal other glands to step up their hormone production. The adrenal glands on top of our kidneys rush adrenaline, cortisol and other hormones into the bloodstream. A cascade of effects is unleashed, including dilated pupils, increased awareness and enhanced reaction time. Digestion slows so that more blood can be diverted to critical organs. Pain tolerance increases and strength is boosted.

When the danger passes, hormone levels return to normal. Under chronic stress, however, the body continues to secrete extra hormones. Over time, they damage organs, muscles and metabolic processes.

The main culprit is cortisol, which has been called the "stress hormone" because of its critical role in chronic stress symptoms. Some cortisol is necessary for good health. Serious deficiency causes Addison's disease and impairs normal brain, immune and muscle function, and disrupts blood circulation. But too much cortisol is just as harmful. Excessive amounts in the body have been linked to an increase in heart rate, blood pressure, and cholesterol and triglyceride levels, making cortisol a risk factor for heart attacks and strokes.[5] Some physicians have called it the most harmful hormone the body produces.[6]

Cortisol compromises the immune system by switching off inflammatory responses that protect our body against infection. Because the nervous system regulates emotional states, it should come as no surprise that cortisol can produce feelings of anxiety, helplessness and pessimism. Excessive amounts of cortisol also can lead to insomnia and loss of sex drive.[7]

In addition, continuous high levels of cortisol can stimulate appetite, resulting in weight gain, obesity and an accumulation of abdominal fat. Other stress reactions include skin conditions such as psoriasis, eczema and acne, and asthma attacks.[8]

The Mental Component

Since so much modern stress has psychological origins, one of the most significant discoveries has been the important role our mind plays as we confront danger. It turns out that in most situations, the way we perceive a threat is much more important than the actual threat itself. In the words of Hans Selye, "It is not stress that kills us, it is our reaction to it."

Because every individual responds to stress differently, what upsets one person may leave another unconcerned or even thrilled. Some people look forward to retirement while others dread it, worrying themselves sick about finances and what to do with themselves. Public speaking may completely unnerve one person, yet it may energize another. Being yelled at by a supervisor can mortify one employee, while another simply shrugs it off.

The difference in our responses to stress may result from early childhood experiences. People who had to endure extreme stress at a young age — domestic violence, divorce, war — tend to be more vulnerable to stress later on in life.[9] There may also be a genetic component to the way we react to stressful situations.

Coping with Stress

In an ideal world, stress management would be part of our daily lives. We would be sure to get eight hours of sleep each night, giving the body time to recover and relax. We would take mini-vacations from work several times a year. We would cultivate stress-reduction techniques such as meditation, massage, biofeedback, yoga and tai chi, especially during times of heightened pressure and tension. And we would develop a positive attitude that would allow us to shrug off many of the things that would otherwise bother us.

Unfortunately, many of us barely manage to practice one or two of these stress management activities and techniques. Instead, many people use negative coping strategies that seem to relieve stress in the short term, but actually compound the problem over time. Abusing alcohol and recreational drugs, smoking cigarettes, and binging on unhealthy foods are common ways people respond to stressful situations.

If you smoke, find a way to quit, whatever it takes. Limit your consumption of alcohol to no more than two glasses a day for men and one glass for women. Also reduce or eliminate coffee, since caffeine aggravates states of tension and anxiety. Many who quit drinking caffeine report sleeping better at night and feeling less agitated during the day.

There are, fortunately, many positive approaches to coping with stress. Here are a few:

BECOME AWARE

Monitor yourself for a week and note what situations cause you distress — deadlines, difficult co-workers, financial challenges. Be sure to include minor irritations. Is it the proverbial toothpaste cap left off or your teenager playing loud rock music? Be specific. Awareness of stress is the first step toward solving the problem.

SHIFT YOUR OUTLOOK

According to Hans Selye, "Adopting the right attitude can convert a negative stress into a positive one." In many cases, simply deciding to look at a situation in a more positive way can reduce the amount of stress in your life. Focus on the opportunities of a difficult situation instead of only the problems. Learn to laugh at yourself and enjoy the comedy of life around you.

CHANGE WHAT YOU CAN

In the morning, many people rush out of the house and feel stressed by the time they get to work. Why not get up half an hour earlier and take your time? Of course, some difficulties may not yield to such simple solutions. If you are stuck in a dead-end job, for example, there may not be a quick fix. But you owe it to yourself to start the process of finding a solution rather than suffering and harming your health.

KEEP BREATHING

The old suggestion to count to 10 and take a deep breath before responding when angry is great wisdom. In the process, we slow down our breathing. Deep breathing is a powerful antidote to stress, which is characterized by short gasps and even holding of the breath.

LEARN TO RELAX

Learn a relaxation technique, such as yoga, meditation or tai chi, and set aside some time each day for practice. Even if you feel you don't have the time, give it a try. You will soon discover that you become more energized and actually gain time because your capacity to get things accomplished grows.

EXERCISE

One of the best ways to burn off stress is to exercise. As Lee Iacocca counsels, "In time of great stress or adversity, it's always best to keep busy and plow your anger and your energy into something positive." Be sure not to overdo it, though.

SHARE YOUR THOUGHTS AND FEELINGS

American men, in particular, grow up learning to keep their feelings to themselves. They consider expressing what bothers them a sign of weakness. We say, on the contrary, it is a sign of courage and maturity. Unburdening yourself to someone else is one of the most effective ways of relieving stress.

GET HELP

It is difficult to break habitual stress patterns on your own. Especially in the case of chronic stress, habitual thoughts and behaviors that trigger stress responses are not easily undone. Psychiatrists, psychologists and other professional counselors are trained to help you break free of these patterns.

Adaptogens

One of the most exciting natural health products to come onto the market in recent years are adaptogens, which can help increase energy and endurance, improve mental alertness, and, above all, reduce the effects of stress on the body. The term "adaptogen" was coined by a Russian scientist, Dr. Nicolai Lazarev, in 1947 to describe medicinal substances with the following characteristics:

- Increase the body's resistance to adverse conditions, such as stress

- Have a normalizing effect on these conditions

- Are safe to use, not affecting the body's normal functions

Lazarev's student, I.I. Brekhman, changed the focus of investigation from synthetic chemical substances to natural substances. He spearheaded the research on several remarkable herbs, including Siberian ginseng (eleuthero) and golden root (rhodiola), and found that they work best in certain combinations.

Since their discovery, these herbs have been tested in more than a thousand clinical studies in Russia and Germany, demonstrating their capacity to strengthen the immune system and reduce stress. The major physiological effects include protection against environmental pollutants, regulation of blood sugar levels, enhancement of the liver's ability to eliminate toxins from the body, an increase in the body's ability to fight infections, and support of optimum adrenal function.

Millions of people in Russia take adaptogens daily, among them sailors and factory workers, to boost their energy and protect themselves against adverse environmental factors. The Russian Olympic team has used adaptogens for decades to reduce stress prior to athletic events and to prevent and treat injuries. Russian cosmonauts have used them to make it easier to adapt to the living conditions in outer space.[10]

Studies have shown the ability of adaptogens to increase resistance to both physical and emotional stress. Unlike drugs, which stimulate the central nervous system, however, adaptogens normalize levels of stress hormones like cortisol, preventing cells and organs from overreacting to stress.[11]

The anti-fatigue properties of adaptogens provide beneficial effects during times of stress and tiredness, making them a better option than pain relief medicine for symptoms of stress, such as headaches, heartburn and indigestion. Available in pill or liquid form, they are an invaluable tool for relieving the effects of chronic stress and improving our health, wellness and longevity.

Getting to Root Causes

Comedian George Burns lived to be 100. When responding to a query about his long life, he said, "If you ask what is the single most important key to longevity, I would have to say it is avoiding worry, stress and tension. And if you didn't ask me, I'd still have to say it."

In today's hustle-and-bustle world, dealing with chronic stress and its debilitating effects is critical. Relaxation strategies and nutritional supplements can help, but to achieve true health and wellness, we have to identify the root causes of stress in our lives and start planting seeds for experiencing joy and pleasure instead.

Three Easy Steps

1. Become aware of all the stress factors in your life.

2. Make the necessary changes in attitude, environment and life style.

3. Take adaptogens on a regular basis.

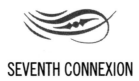

SEVENTH CONNEXION

A BALANCED LIFE

---

*I've learned that you can't have everything
and do everything at the same time.*

OPRAH WINFREY

Most people complain of not having enough time. They feel
overwhelmed by all the demands at work and at home. Most
parents with children younger than 18 work outside the home.
As our population ages, many men and women work as well
as take care of children and their aging parents. With a host of
responsibilities tugging at them from all sides, they have little
time for doing even such ordinary activities as cleaning the house
and cooking meals, much less exercising, pursuing hobbies and
spending time with each other.

As a result, they feel overwhelmed, overtired and overstressed.
With no relief in sight, they become exhausted, anxious, irritable
and depressed. Relationships suffer from neglect, work becomes a
chore, and life becomes a drudgery. They don't have fun with their
partners or children. Downtime and "me time" have become distant
memories of a golden past.

No wonder many people yearn for balance in their lives.

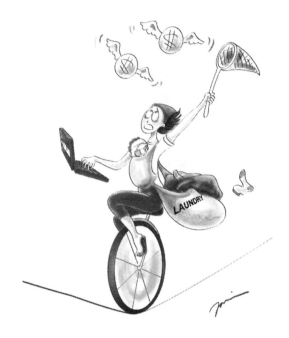

Modern, multi-tasking Mom

Everyone feels overwhelmed at times — during a crisis or when the demands of everyday life build up. Stress is okay as long as it passes soon and equilibrium is restored; but when it becomes a chronic condition, its effect on physical and mental health and wellness is harmful. Chances are, if you are feeling stress on a daily basis for two or more weeks, you are desperately in need of a way to restore your balance.

Why is it essential to regain your equilibrium? Because if you do not, burnout looms around the corner.

What to Do?

The first step is to realize that you are in control of your life to a much greater degree than you probably think you are.

Next, make the decision to have a more balanced life.

Most people live in reaction to outside demands and events, bobbing from crisis to crisis like a boat in a storm-tossed sea. Few drop anchor, take charge and design their lives, which is essential to achieving balance and well-being. The decisions you make, pursued consistently over time, will become what you achieve in life. What you accomplish is the sum total of all the decisions you make. You do not determine your success. You determine your daily habits, and they shape your success.

If you don't take charge, you may never have the opportunity to realize your potential. Even if you are successful, you may feel unfulfilled because you have focused exclusively on one aspect of what could have been a multi-faceted life. If you only work, or only go to the gym, or only watch TV, you may miss out on all of life's pleasures and possibilities. Don't let life just happen to you.

Of course there are times when your life is going to be "out of whack." Sometimes you have to be out of balance for a season, if there is a crisis — a deadline at work, a sick child at home, a parent going into the hospital. But you do not have to stay stuck in crisis mode forever.

Hurdles and Obstacles to Balanced Living

Many people would love to live a more balanced life but don't know how. Having to deal with stressful situations too much of the time, they become habitually overwhelmed. It is nearly impossible to reinvent the wheel while you are busy pushing it.

The first thing to do is to stop, take stock of where you are, and get ready to make some changes. As with every wellness principle we have discussed so far, living a balanced life is a process and will require some time and attention. Remember, if you don't take charge of your life, others will make all the decisions for you, and stress will result from lack of control.

We recommend a four-step approach to busy-ness as usual:

1. Decide what truly matters to you.

2. Prioritize according to your values.

3. Put your priorities on a monthly schedule.

4. Follow through.

What Truly Matters to You

Start by listing all the things that are important to you. These may include family, faith, fitness, finances, friends; pets, food, sports and personal growth. Because most of us are not used to thinking this way, we suggest that you brainstorm and give yourself the freedom to include things you normally would not consider except in your wildest dreams. Be sure to not limit yourself to the tasks you know you have to do; include the things you want to do for yourself, even if they have been beyond your reach up to now.

Prioritize

Pick the five most important items from your list, the five areas in your life that you value most and really care about. Many people think of values as broad, unchanging categories like integrity, love and honesty. But unlike principles, which are eternal, values can vary with time, depending on your experiences, interests and stages of life. Cars and pizza are more important to many male teenagers than to their adult counterparts. A married graduate student may care only about her studies and her husband; but when children enter the picture, her values will change considerably. As Bill Gates said, "In my 20s, I worked very, very hard. I have a much more balanced life now."

As an example, here is a list of the top five most important areas in our lives. Yours may be different.

Faith

Family

Fitness

Finance

Personal Growth

FAITH

We believe that we are created by a loving God, who has a purpose and plan for each of our lives. Cultivating an ever-deepening relationship with our creator is a vital part of a fulfilling life.

FAMILY

Scheduling time to be with your spouse, children and extended family can help assure that you are giving them the attention they deserve. One of the authors, for example, schedules time to be with his wife. It is important to him — he has realized that he tends to be active, busy and preoccupied — and if he did not deliberately make the time and effort, it would not happen.

FITNESS

Exercising mind and body was as important to the ancient Greeks as it is today. Physical, mental, and emotional vitality are essential for a successful, balanced life. Fitness leads to health, wellness and peace of mind.

FINANCE

Planning long-term financial goals, learning to become debt free, building an investment portfolio or owning businesses — decide what truly matters to you and schedule the time to devote to it. Most people barely make it to the end of the month on their money, which causes financial pressure.

PERSONAL GROWTH

It was Socrates who said, "An unexamined life is not worth living." Growing and changing can occur throughout one's life. Reading books, listening to tapes or CDs, attending seminars, pursuing hobbies, visiting museums, attending concerts, learning languages, acquiring new skills, traveling, meeting new people — there are many ways to grow.

If your list includes areas that have not been a part of your life up to now, it is critical that you figure out how to make the necessary changes to include them. Why end your life's journey with bitterness and regret instead of a sense of accomplishment and fulfillment?

Schedule

This is the stumbling block for most people. PDAs, organizers and to-do lists can get you through the day, but they may not be that helpful to getting your life in balance.

Take a monthly calendar and first block out tasks you must do and activities beyond your control. If you have a job that requires you to work eight hours a day, you don't control that time. But you can be in charge of the other 16 hours a day and the weekends.

Take the first item on your list and block out time for it in your schedule. Then do the second item and so on. Include broad strokes and detailed subcategories. Family may involve time for activities with children like a son's basketball games, or helping with homework and time with your spouse. Make sure you include time alone together. If you have children, get a sitter or trade with other couples for time off.

Be sure to schedule downtime for rest and relaxation. Not only will you enjoy and appreciate life more fully, but you are likely to discover that you become more productive in the other areas of your life. As Ovid, the Latin poet, recommended 2,000 years ago, "Take rest. A field that has rested gives a bountiful crop."

You will find that experience teaches you how much or little time each activity requires. So when you first start, monitor your progress and be prepared to make adjustments. In time, making a schedule based on your values and priorities will become easier. While you may chafe at feeling restricted, trust that the process will liberate rather than limit you. In any designated block of time, whether it involves work, sleep or fun, you have the freedom to be 100 percent focused on a scheduled activity without any feeling any guilt.

Follow Through

Actually doing what you schedule is a challenging part of balancing your life. But with a list of priorities and a schedule based on what matters to you, you have a tool to evaluate and respond to what is important. It makes no sense to give up a number one or two priority time slot for a number four or lower demand. If family is your top priority and a friend or business associate needs to see you when you are scheduled to watch your son's baseball game or your daughter's dance recital, you do not need to feel torn. If fitness is high on your list, you no longer need to interrupt your exercise in order to take a phone call. You have a clear road map of priorities.

Learn to Say "No"

Most important is learning to say "no" to the people who want to take your time, and to the things that people want you to do. Let others handle some of what you don't want to do. Do not make commitments just because you think you have to.

It may take some practice to get past the initial feeling of discomfort, especially for people who are used to saying "yes" to everyone who asks them to do something. Taking on too many commitments is stressful and makes it impossible to live a balanced life. Let someone else run the school fund-raiser this year. Pass on a new project at work when you have too many duties already. Imagine the pleasure of being able to cross items off your list because you have developed the ability to say "no."

In some cases, you may need to get creative about removing items from your to-do list. Consider delegating some chores to other family members. If you can afford it, hire someone to clean your home, do the yard work or make minor repairs. Start your holiday shopping early. Imagine the decrease in pressure if you finish your Christmas list by Labor Day!

Unloading extra projects does mean giving up control and admitting to yourself that many things can and will happen without you. But the benefits will be huge.

Don't Expect to be Perfect

Don't be too hard on yourself when you go off your schedule. As with exercising and any of the other principles, resist an "all or nothing" attitude. No one follows a plan 100 percent all the time. Remind yourself that you are human, laugh at yourself, and reaffirm your commitment. Stay the course.

There will be times when you have no choice but to go off your schedule. Life-threatening events and emergencies always take priority. But even during those times, your priority list will allow you to make better judgments about what you can leave undone and what you must take care of.

Reward Yourself

An important aspect of achieving balance is to reward yourself for successfully completing incremental goals. If you manage to keep doing the things on your schedule, you are accomplishing more than most ever do. So rejoice. Buy yourself a present. Treat yourself.

The point is that the process never ends. Like a gymnast on a balance beam, maintaining your equilibrium takes determination and constant adjusting. Whenever you reach a milestone, you owe it to yourself to celebrate.

Three Easy Steps

1. Decide to live a more balanced life.

2. Make a list of your priorities and schedule them on a monthly basis.

3. Follow through and reward yourself when you succeed.

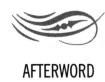

AFTERWORD

THE NEXT STEP

---

*Wisdom is knowing what to do, skill is knowing
how to do it, and virtue is doing it.*

DAVID STARR JORDAN, AMERICAN EDUCATOR

Knowing and doing are two different things. All the knowledge about carbs and calories will not trim one ounce of fat from your body. Understanding the principle of pure water will not prevent you from being the filter and repository for environmental toxins. Now it is time to take action. The way to truly know about healthy living is to make it part of your everyday life.

Our bodies may be designed for living 125 years, but if we don't take care of them, they will rust, sputter and break down like a car that does not receive proper maintenance. Regular upkeep is essential for a long, healthy life.

Professional athletes and other high-level performers know the importance of taking care of themselves. They train every day to keep their bodies in shape, their "instrument" in tune. As Sandy Koufax, the Hall of Fame baseball pitcher once said, "People who write about spring training not being necessary have never tried to throw a baseball."

While you may not perform at the level of an athletic superstar or a concert pianist, the process is the same for living a full, energetic life and enjoying your work, family, friends, hobbies and recreation. It takes practice, practice, practice. In the words of the ancient Greek sage Periander: "Practice is everything."

Our Challenge to You

We challenge you to take the next step on your life's journey and make the most of these wellness conneXions. Make a decision to take charge of your life and pursue a healthy existence. Then, set some priorities and goals, and make time for them. Put them in your schedule. The time you spend practicing the seven principles will return to you tenfold.

We urge you to commit yourself to make at least one conneXion a month for each of the seven principles. Some may be simple to accomplish, for example, purchasing a sports bottle or taking a daily multivitamin. Others, such as avoiding sugars and other high glycemic carbohydrates or getting on an exercise program, may be more challenging.

Whatever the case, take that first step and then another and another. Expect to stumble once in a while, and even to have to backtrack from time to time. You don't have to be perfect. You just need to keep going. In the process, positive changes and unexpected surprises will happen. What Arnold Palmer said about golf applies to the pursuit of health and wellness, too: "It's a funny thing, the more I practice, the luckier I get."

So get going. Start integrating these principles into your daily life. And, above all, take all the pleasure you can along the way, have fun with the process, and enjoy the journey.

We wish you Ageless Vitality in the years ahead.

REFERENCES

Introduction

1. United Health Foundation, "America's Health: State Health Rankings — 2004 Edition."

2. American Obesity Association (AOA), 2002.

3. "Diabetes Statistics for Youth," American Diabetes Association, www.diabetes.org.

4. "Pharmacist Organization Unveils Snapshot of Medication Use in U.S.," American Society of Health-System Pharmacists, January 16, 2001.

5. "The Pharmaceutical Market," Association of Research-based Pharmaceutical Companies, VFA ©2005.

6. Paul Zane Pilzer, *The Wellness Revolution*, John Wiley & Sons: NJ: 2002.

7. Ibid.

8. Mike Adams, "One-third of Americans diet is junk food and soft drinks: we're malnourished and obese at the same time," www.newstarget.com, June 2, 2002.

9. The Greenlining Institute, press release, December 23, 2002, www.greenling.org.

10. John Castaldo, M.D., et al., "Physician Attitudes Regarding Cardiovascular Risk Reduction: The Gaps Between Clinical Importance, Knowledge, and Effectiveness," Disease Management, April 2005, Vol. 8, No. 2: 93-105.

11. "Processed Foods," www.mcvitamins.com, 2000-2005.

12. Sherry A. Rogers, M.D., *Detoxify or Die*, Sand Key Company, Inc, Sarasota: 2002.

13. Florence Williams, "Toxic Breast Milk?", New York Times Magazine, January 9, 2005.

14. Sherry A. Rogers, *Detoxify or Die.*

15. American Academy of Anti-Aging Medicine, www.worldhealth.net.

16. "The Politics of Food: A Brief History of the U.S. Dietary Guidelines," Physicians Committee for responsible Medicine, 2000.

Chapter 1: Pure Water

1. "Dishonorable Discharge: Toxic Pollution of America's Water," Environmental Working Group (EWG) Report, September 1996.

2. USA Today, June 1999.

3. "Troubled Waters on Tap: Organic Chemicals in Public Drinking Water Systems and the Failure of Regulation," Center for Study of Responsive Law (Ralph Nader's Organization), 1988.

4. NBC Nightly News as aired on October 5, 2004.

5. "Is Your Water Safe," US News & World Report, July 29, 1991.

6. Payment, P. et al., "A Randomized Trial to Evaluate the Risk of Gastrointestinal Disease Due to Consumption of Drinking Water Meeting Current Microbial Standards," American Journal of Public Health, June 1991, vol. 81, no. 6, pp. 703-708.

7. Joseph M. Price, *Coronaries/Colesterouchlorine*, Jove Books, Alta Enterprises: 1969.

8. Dons Bach KW, M. Walker, "Drinking Water," Huntingdon Beach, CA: International Institute of Natural Health Sciences, 1981.

9. Ian Anderson, "Showers Pose a Risk to Health," New Scientist, November 19, 1986.

10. Lance A. Wallace, "Human Exposure to Volatile Organic Pollutants: Implications for Indoor Air Studies," Annual Review of Energy and the Environment, November 2001.

11. "Bottled Water: Pure Drink or Pure Hype?", National Research Defense Council (NDRC), March 1999.

12. John Stossel, "Is Bottled Water Better than Tap?", ABC News Internet Ventures, 2005.

13. Ibid.

14. Judith Valentine, "The Dangers of Soft Drinks - America," Global Healing Center news letter, January 8, 2003.

Chapter 2: Eating Well

1. "Dieting and the Diet Industry," National Association to Advance fat Acceptance, May 30, 1993.

2. "The Politics of Food: A Brief History of the U.S. Dietary Guidelines," Physicians Committee for responsible Medicine, 2000.

3. Lisa Greene, "Food Pyramid History," December 2, 2002.

4. Erasmus, Udo, Ph.D., *Fats that Heal, Fats that Kill*, Alive Books: 1987, 1993.

5. Finnegan, John, N.D., *The Facts About Fats*, Celestial Arts Publishing: 1993.

6. Michio Kushi, with Stephen Blauer, *The Macrobiotic Way: The Complete Macrobiotic Diet and Exercise Book*, Penguin Group (USA): 1993.

7. Graham Simpson, M.D., Stephen T. Sinatra, M.D. & Jorge Suárez-Menéndez, M.D., *Spa Medicine: Your Gateway to the Ageless Zone*, Basic Health Publications, Inc.: 2004.

8. Judith Valentine, "The Dangers of Soft Drinks - America," Global Healing Center news letter, January 8, 2003.

9. Paul Zane Pilzer, *The Wellness Revolution*, John Wiley & Sons: NJ: 2002.

10. Karen Collins, R.D., "More Good News about the Mediterranean Diet," special to MSNBC, October 29, 2004.

11. Rita Mae Brown, *Starting from Scratch*, Bantam Books, 1988.

Chapter 3: Eliminating Toxins

1. Sherry A. Rogers, M.D., *Detoxify or Die*, Sand Key Company, Inc, Sarasota: 2002.

2. Ibid.

3. Ibid.

4. Ibid.

5. Nicholas A. Ashford and Claudia S. Miller, "Low-Level Chemical Exposures: A Challenge for Science and Policy, Viewpoint, November 1, 1998 / Volume 32, Issue 21.

6. "Body Burden2: The Pollution in Newborns: Human Health Problems on the Rise," EWG Report, July 14, 2005.

7. Sherry A. Rogers, *Detoxify or Die.*

8. Graham Simpson, M.D., Stephen T. Sinatra, M.D. & Jorge Suárez-Menéndez, M.D., *Spa Medicine: Your Gateway to the Ageless Zone*, Basic Health Publications, Inc.: 2004.

9. John Emsley, *Elements of Murder: A History of Poison*, Oxford University Press: 2005.

10. "Body Burden2."

11. "Toxic Bodies are a Bad Sign: Kid's Health Especially at Risk," Editorial, Ventura County star, August 7, 2005.

12. Gary A. Davis and Em Turner, "Safe Substitutes at Home: Non-Toxic Household Products," University of Tennessee - Knoxville Waste Management Institute Working Paper.

13. Susan Yara, "The Best (Worst) Foods," Forbes.com.

14. "Shopper's Guide to Pesticides in Produce," Food News, EWG, October 21, 2003.

15. Sherry A. Rogers, *Detoxify or Die.*

16. "Dental Amalgam Controversy," Wikipedia, the free encyclopedia.

17. Sherry A. Rogers, *Detoxify or Die.*

Chapter 4: Supplementation

1. Robert M. Russell and Joel B. Mason, "The Graying of Society: Nutrition, Vitamins and Aging, www.thedoctorwillseeyounow.com, April 2000.

2. "Minerals," www.1HealthyWorld.com, Library of health, ©LLC, 2003.

3. "Vitamin supplements and why we need them," What Doctors Don't Tell You Magazine, December 2002.

4. "Processed Foods," wwwmcvitamins.com, 2000-2005.

5. "Vitamins & Aging," www.healthbulletin.org.

6. Robert M. Russel, et al., "The Graying of Society."

7. Ibid.

8. "Recommended Dietary Allowances," Subcommittee of the Tenth Edition of the RDAs. Food and Nutrition Board Commission on Life Sciences. National Research Council:, 10th edition, Washington, DC: National Academy Press: Summary Table, 1989.

9. Donald Rudin, MD, and Clara Felix, *Omega-3 Oils: A Practical Guide*, US: Avery, 1996.

10. "Lycopene: an Antioxidant for Good Health," American Dietetic Association, © 2002.

11. In a 1995 Harvard University study conducted with 47,894 men, researchers found that eating 10 or more servings a week of tomato products was associated with a reduced risk of prostate cancer by as much as 34 percent.

12. Daniel Rudman, M.D., et al., "Effects of human Growth Hormone in Men over 60 Years Old," New England Journal of Medicine, Volume 323, Number 1, July 5, 1990.

Chapter 6: Exercising

1. "Top 500 Franchises List," Entrepreneur's Magazine.

2. Durstine J.L. & W.L. Haskell, "Effects of Exercise Training on Plasma Lipids and Lipoproteins," Exercise and Sports Science Reviews. 1994, 22:477-522.

3. "Why Should I be Physically Active," American Heart Association, 2004.

4. Loretta DiPietro, Phd, MPH; James Dziura, MPH, "Exercise: A Prescription to Delay the Effects of Aging," The Physician and Sports Medicine, Vol. 28, No. 10, October 2000.

5. University of Michigan Health System M-Fit Health Promotion Division, April 2004.

6. Cenegenics Medical Institute Patient Guide.

7. Ibid.

8. "Stretching, Strengthening Ease Chronic Back Pain," Reuters Health, May 2, 2005.

9. "If You're Fat, It Doesn't Matter if You're Fit," Reuters Health April 19, 2005.

Chapter 6: Stress Management

1. Simpson, Sinatra, Suárez-Menéndez, *Spa Medicine*, Basic Health Publications: 2004.

2. Atkinson R.L. et al, *Hilgard's Introduction to Psychology*, 1996.

3. Herbert Benson, M.D, Julie Corliss and Geoffrey Cowley, "Brain Check," Newsweek, September 27, 2004.

4. "The Different Kinds of Stress," American Psychological Association, APA Help Center, 2004.

5. "Stress: Why your have it and how it hurts your health," MayoClinic.com, September 17, 2004.

6. Simpson, Sinatra, Suárez-Menéndez, *Spa Medicine*.

7. Ibid., "Stress: Why you have it."

8. James South, M.A., "Stress and Cortisol: The Plague of the 21st Century," Vitamin Research Products, vpr.com/art/1224.asp.

9. "The Different Kinds of Stress."

10. Christopher Hobbs, L.A.C., A.H.G., "Herbal Adaptogens Fitting Into The Modern Age," HealthWorld Online (www.healthy.net) 1996.

11. A. Panossian, *Adaptogens*, Alternative & Complementary Therapies," December 2003, 327-331.

ABOUT THE AUTHORS

Dan Watts, M.D.

Dr. Watts has practiced medicine and surgery for more than 30 years. A Fellow of the American College of Surgeons and the American College of Obstetrics and Gynecology, Dr. Watts is listed in "Best Doctors in America." He has held an appointment as clinical professor at the University of South Florida College of Medicine.

As a family practitioner and gynecologist, Dr. Watts discovered that a number of his patients suffered aging-related problems such as hormone imbalances and osteoporosis. Knowing that these conditions are both preventable and curable, he embarked on a rigorous study of the aging process and its effects on general health. He is one of only 1,000 doctors worldwide to be Board Certified by the American Academy of Anti-Aging Medicine. He is Founder and Director of The Renewal Point Anti-Aging Center in Sarasota, Florida, which includes a full service Med Spa.

His wife, Sherry, has worked side by side with him in founding The Renewal Point. Their daughter, Ashlee, holds a Masters of Science Degree in Public Health and is the Program Director of the Campus Wellness Center at the University of South Carolina. Their son, Danny, attends Florida State University, majoring in finance and economics. Dr. Watts has a passion for off-road bicycling, and hits the trails on weekends whenever he can. He follows all of the wellness principles in this book and admits to having difficulties with eating right. While the food he eats is healthful most of the time, consuming it in moderation is his challenge (www.therenewalpoint.com).

Adrian Lewis, M.D.

Dr. Lewis was born in London, England. After graduating from medical school at the University of Cape Town in South Africa, he and his wife, Sue, a physical therapist, came to the United States and settled in Gainesville, Florida, where he has been a family physician since 1982 (www.lewishhealthcare.com).

During the 1990s, Dr. Lewis also built an international marketing company that sold wellness products, including nutritional supplements, water filtration systems and skin care products. He is the co-founder of a national company that promotes wellness communities. He is also co-founder of Wellness ConneXion, LLC, and Haile Wellness Club (www.HaileWellnessClub.com), dedicated to connecting wellness providers and consumers.

Faith and family are very important to Dr. Lewis. He has two sons — Andrew, a sophomore at the University of Florida, and Mathew, a junior in high school. Dr. Lewis loves to travel. In the last year, he was a member of a medical mission team to China. He also visited South Africa, Turkey, Italy and the Greek Isles. He follows all the recommendations in this book, but acknowledges that, although he lives a balanced life, his biggest challenge remains getting enough rest, because he never seems to have enough time to fit in all of his interests and commitments into a 24-hour day.

Steve Kalishman, J.D.

Steve Kalishman received degrees in journalism and law from the University of Florida. Since 1982, he has been practicing law throughout Florida in state and federal trial and appellate courts, with a focus on medical issues involving traumatic injuries. A resident of Gainesville since 1970, he is the Founding Director of sister programs between Gainesville and Novorossiisk, Russia, and Kfar Saba/Qalqilya in Israel (www.GnvSisterCities.org). While working as a cook on a merchant ship, he met and married his wife, Natalia, in Russia in 1976. They have a 16-year-old bilingual daughter, and they practice law together at Steven Kalishman, PA, law office (www.FlaLitiGators.com).

As a founder/partner of Transamerica Marketing, Inc., Steve has been lecturing about the importance of nutritional supplements, water filters, skin care products and a balanced lifestyle for the past 15 years. He is also co-founder of Wellness ConneXion, LLC, and Haile Wellness Club (www.HaileWellnessClub.com), dedicated to connecting wellness providers and consumers.

Because he is a passionate gourmet cook, he has the most difficulty with eating right. He finds it especially difficult to resist bread and pasta. To compensate for his weaknesses, he utilizes strategies such as drinking plenty of pure water and keeping fruit and other healthful snacks around the house. He enjoys biking, golf and travel.

For more information visit our Web site at
www.wellnessconnexion.com